Evaluation of the Psychiatric Patient

A PRIMER

CRITICAL ISSUES IN PSYCHIATRY
An Educational Series for Residents and Clinicians

Series Editor: Sherwyn M. Woods, M.D., Ph.D.
University of Southern California School of Medicine
Los Angeles, California

Recent volumes in the series:

CASE STUDIES IN INSOMNIA
Edited by Peter J. Hauri

CLINICAL DISORDERS OF MEMORY
Aman U. Khan, M.D.

CONTEMPORARY PERSPECTIVES ON PSYCHOTHERAPY WITH
LESBIANS AND GAY MEN
Edited by Terry S. Stein, M.D., and Carol J. Cohen, M.D.

DIAGNOSTIC AND LABORATORY TESTING IN PSYCHIATRY
Edited by Mark S. Gold, M.D., and A. L. C. Pottash, M.D.

DRUG AND ALCOHOL ABUSE: A Clinical Guide to Diagnosis
and Treatment, Third Edition
Marc A. Schuckit, M.D.

EMERGENCY PSYCHIATRY: Concepts, Methods, and Practices
Edited by Ellen L. Bassuk, M.D., and Ann W. Birk, Ph.D.

ETHNIC PSYCHIATRY
Edited by Charles B. Wilkinson, M.D.

EVALUATION OF THE PSYCHIATRIC PATIENT: A Primer
Seymour L. Halleck

NEUROPSYCHIATRIC FEATURES OF MEDICAL DISORDERS
James W. Jefferson, M.D., and John R. Marshall, M.D.

THE RACE AGAINST TIME: Psychotherapy and Psychoanalysis
in the Second Half of Life
Edited by Robert A. Nemiroff, M.D., and Calvin A. Colarusso, M.D.

STATES OF MIND: Configurational Analysis of Individual
Psychology, Second Edition
Mardi J. Horowitz, M.D.

A Continuation Order Plan is available for this series. A continuation order will bring
delivery of each new volume immediately upon publication. Volumes are billed only upon
actual shipment. For further information please contact the publisher.

Evaluation of the Psychiatric Patient

A PRIMER

Seymour L. Halleck

University of North Carolina
Chapel Hill, North Carolina

Plenum Medical Book Company • New York and London

Library of Congress Cataloging in Publication Data

Halleck, Seymour L.
  Evaluation of the psychiatric patient: a primer / Seymour L. Halleck.
    p.   cm.—(Critical issues in psychiatry)
  Includes bibliographical references and index.
  ISBN 978-1-4684-5882-4
  1. Interviewing in psychiatry. 2. Mental illness—Diagnosis. I. Title. II. Series.
  [DNLM: 1. Interview, Psychological. 2. Mental Disorders—diagnosis. WM 141
H164e]
  RC480.7.H35   1991
  616.89′075—dc20
  DNLM/DLC   90-14351
  for Library of Congress   CIP

ISBN 978-1-4684-5882-4   ISBN 978-1-4684-5880-0 (eBook)
DOI 10.1007/978-1-4684-5880-0

© 1991 Plenum Publishing Corporation
Softcover reprint of the hardcover 1st edition 1991
233 Spring Street, New York, N.Y. 10013

Plenum Medical Book Company is an imprint of Plenum Publishing Corporation

Preface

A few months before the final manuscript of this book was sent to the publisher, Dr. Karl A. Menninger died, shortly before his ninety-seventh birthday. Thus, when I sat down to write this preface, he was very much on my mind. I remembered that it had been almost forty years since he wrote *A Manual for Psychiatric Case Study*, not one of his well-known but probably the most practical of his books. The psychoanalytically trained part of me began to wonder what had motivated me to write a book on a topic so similar to that which had earlier drawn the attention of my revered teacher. There is no pressing need for another book on psychiatric evaluation; furthermore, evaluation is a very difficult subject to write about in a straightforward way.

Whatever my unconscious motivations may have been, I hope they were less significant than those of which I was aware. I wrote this book mainly as part of an effort to reverse certain trends in psychiatric education. In the last decade psychiatrists have increasingly been trained in an environment that emphasizes brief evaluation of patients and de-emphasizes teaching about the complexity of human behavior and experience. Trainees no longer study psychiatric evaluation in a systematic manner. They take fewer intensive histories, fill out forms instead of describing the patient's mental status, and, with rare exceptions, are not taught how to conceptualize biological and psychosocial interactions.

One need only compare a hospital chart of a decade ago with a current one to realize what has been lost. The modern chart tends to be more perfect from a legalistic and utilization review standpoint. In contrast to the older chart, it is likely to have fewer missing notations, without failure to record interventions. What is missing from the modern chart, however, is a description of a person. One could search through its pages and find almost nothing about how the patient has lived his or her life, or how the tragedy of mental illness has influenced that life and that of the patient's loved ones. Nor can one learn very much about the patient's personality, other than what is too often a pejorative use of a *DSM-III-R* Axis II label. What has in the past been variously described as a humanistic, existential, holistic, multidimensional or systems-oriented approach to evaluation and treatment is in danger of disappearing.

I believe that the current reductionistic approach to psychiatry, whether driven by cost-containment, new biological discoveries, or new categorical approaches to diagnosis, is bad for our patients. Too often, it leads to under-diagnosis, over-diagnosis, or inaccurate diagnosis followed by inappropriate and sometimes harmful treatment.

This book can be viewed as a plea for students to approach psychiatric evaluation with a healthy reverence for the complexity and difficulty of the task. It calls upon the student to examine all dimensions of the patient's personhood, from biological to spiritual. Because it is not reductionistic, its mastery may require more effort on the part of the reader than other texts on this subject. Hopefully, this effort will be more than compensated for, if the student can discover or rediscover the emotional and intellectual joys of dealing with a patient in all dimensions of personhood.

In a sense, this is an old-fashioned book, conveying the message that some, but certainly not all, of the old ways are better. The book is not intended to present new ideas, but rather to synthesize old ones and to show how they are relevant to modern technologies. Whatever might be found here that is original is a description of my own techniques in evaluating patients and some ideas I have developed about evaluating patients' capacities through my forensic work.

I have no illusions that this book will have a significant impact on how psychiatry is practiced. The forces influencing modern psychiatry, particularly economic forces, are powerful and a single treatise on evaluation is unlikely to diminish them. Yet, one must act on what one believes and hope that it will have some influence on those beginning the study of this very exciting profession. As I write this, I cannot help wishing that Dr. Menninger were still around to make the case for humanistic psychiatry in a manner of which I am not capable. His genius, his eloquence, and his influence are sorely missed.

Many people helped me with this book. Laura Deiulio, Alane Hare, and Mary Lou Allison were diligent and patient in typing the many drafts of the text. Ken Selig, Sean Shea, Sherwyn Woods, Jeffry Andresen, and Joseph Noschpitz read earlier drafts and provided very helpful commentary. Joe, in his characteristic, loving way, sent back the manuscript with line by line editing, a gift I deeply appreciate.

Contents

Contents

The Problems of Evaluation in Psychiatry

When residents and medical students begin to work with psychiatric patients, they have already learned a great deal about the process of medical evaluation. They know how to detect signs and symptoms of illness by taking a history and performing a physical examination. They have also learned how to use abnormal findings as a guide to laboratory testing and to appreciate the relevance of these findings to diagnosis and treatment. These skills are all necessary or essential in treating psychiatric patients. Unfortunately, they are far from sufficient.

Unlike other medical specialties, in which training is built almost entirely on an expansion of learning processes already initiated in medical school, psychiatric training requires the student to master perspectives, skills, and knowledge that have not previously been taught. As a result, psychiatric residents experience more difficulty in making the transition from medical student to resident than do residents in other specialties, and medical students are frequently confused and discouraged by the seemingly foreign nature of the psychiatric rotation.

Many of the difficulties of learning to be a psychiatrist are ultimately determined by subtle but fundamental differences between mental and physical illnesses. The traditional pedagogical approach in psychiatry is to encourage students to ignore or minimize these differences and to emphasize the similarities between all illnesses. Although this emphasis is reassuring to students, it can also retard or inhibit their capacity to grapple with issues that are critical to psychiatric management and treatment. The approach here is to acknowledge the similarities between physical and mental illness but also to focus on those differences that have a direct influence on the process of psychiatric evaluation.

HOW DOES THE MANNER IN WHICH
MENTAL ILLNESSES ARE DEFINED INFLUENCE
THE PROCESS OF PSYCHIATRIC EVALUATION?

Psychiatric disorders (in the course of this discussion the terms *illness, disease,* and *disorder* will be used interchangeably) are defined and classified primarily on the basis of observations of the patient's behavior and experience. Almost all of the diagnostic criteria listed in the revised third edition of the American Psychiatric Association's *Diagnostic and Statistical Manual* (DSM-III-R; APA, 1987) can be viewed as either an aberration of behavior or as some abnormality of inner (or subjective) experience (of perceiving, thinking, or feeling). The DSM-III-R diagnostic criteria for major depressive episodes are typical and illustrative. They include:

1. Depressed mood (an experiential [subjective] criterion).
2. Diminished interest in activities (experiential).
3. Significant weight loss or weight gain (an outcome of behavior that in turn may be related to the experience of change in appetite).
4. Insomnia or hypersomnia (behavioral).
5. Psychomotor agitation or retardation (behavioral).
6. Fatigue or loss of energy (experiential).
7. Feelings of worthlessness or excessive or inappropriate guilt (experiential).
8. Diminished ability to think or concentrate or indecisiveness (experiential).
9. Recurrent thoughts of death or suicidal ideation (experiential) or a suicide attempt (behavioral).

Atypical behavior and/or experience may also be part of the presentation of physical illness. Almost all patients show some type of help-seeking behavior, some patients curtail their activities, and most complain about unpleasant internal experiences such as pain, dizziness, or fatigue. The emphasis in defining physical illness, however, is on uncovering and measuring characteristic anatomical and physiological changes in organ systems, and the patient's atypical behavior and experience are assumed to be appropriate responses to those pathophysiological changes.

In psychiatry, the patient's behavioral and experiential symptoms are in themselves viewed as inappropriate and pathological. Psychiatrists increasingly seek to relate these behavioral and experiential findings to organic dysfunction. The range of abnormal behavior and experience is so great, however, that often it is not possible to relate specific symptoms to specific biological changes. Even when organic causes of mental conditions become more carefully defined, the accuracy of psychiatric diagnosis is still likely to be determined by the thoroughness and precision with which symptoms are assessed. It is the need to make a proper assessment of behavioral and experiential symptoms that requires the physician to develop new perspectives and skills.

When evaluating behavioral manifestations of mental disorders, the psychiatrist must acquire several skills, namely, how to obtain accurate descriptions of abnormal behavior from the patient or other observers, and how to make direct observations of the patient's current behavior. Some patients are able to describe troubling aspects of their own behavior with relative clarity. Others, however, cannot. More objective accounts of the patient's aberrant behavior are likely to be obtained from the patient's family, friends, or others who have interacted with him or her. Sometimes, the physician is concerned with behavior, such as inappropriate aggressivity or withdrawal, that is viewed as pathological or deviant either by the patient or by others. At other times, the physician is concerned with a behavioral abnormality that is characterized by a deficit in functioning or by the patient's apparent lack of ability to accomplish tasks that were once accomplished more easily. In any case, assessment of behavioral abnormality routinely requires a considerable amount of history taking to determine past patterns of behavior. The psychiatrist must be concerned with how long the behavioral aberrations have been present, whether they have occurred previously, and how much the current behavior differs from the patient's usual patterns of conduct.

It is also critical that the clinician develop skills in detecting current behavioral aberrations, in particular, patterns that are likely to appear during the process of evaluation. To develop such skills the psychiatrist must extend his or her medical observational capacities and learn to be a participant observer who is constantly aware of how the patient interacts with her or him throughout each interview. Skills are also required in observing how patients behave in their interactions with other patients, with hospital staff, and with family members.

The task of learning about and describing the patient's experiences is more complex. Thoughts, feelings, and perceptions are private phenomena, and many patients are unwilling or unable to discuss them with the physician. One of the first skills that a psychiatrist must master is how to ask questions about inner experiences that patients can understand and answer. The psychiatrist must also learn how to establish a professional relationship with patients that allows them to feel sufficient trust so that they are willing to share the nature of their experience.

Sometimes, the nature of the patient's present experience can be elucidated by focusing on the past. By developing an accurate history of what experiences patients have had in past environments, the psychiatrist may be able to infer something about how they may be experiencing their current environment. To make these kinds of inferences, the psychiatrist must be skilled in taking a detailed history of past experience.

Even when patients are interviewed skillfully, their communications may be inaccurate or distorted. The psychiatrist must, therefore, develop competence in determining when patients are presenting misleading information. When information supplied by the patient is insufficient or inaccurate, the psychiatrist can seek more detailed and accurate information about certain internal experiences by asking questions that test the patient's perceptual and thought processes. These questions form part of the traditional mental status examination; they often reveal evidences of pathology that the patient would not or could not describe in an ordinary conversation.

In psychiatry, the issue of the accuracy with which the patient reports or reveals experience is especially critical. When the nature of internal experience is part of the definition of a mental disorder, the accuracy of diagnosis is directly correlated with the accuracy of the patient's reporting. Yet, the possibilities of inaccurate reporting are very high. There are many reasons for psychiatric patients to exaggerate, minimize, or just lie about their symptoms. Fear of mental illness, concern about stigmatization, wishes for more attention, or some form of excuse from responsibility often leads to inaccurate reporting. It is also very difficult for the physician to assess the accuracy of patient reporting; at best, it is rarely possible to detect physiological abnormalities that explain and confirm the patient's reported experience.

Finally, the psychiatrist must be concerned with the relationship of the patient's behavior and experience. In some instances, inner experience can be inferred by observing deviant patterns of behavior. The patient who is withdrawn and tearful is likely to feel sad. In other situations, behavior may be predicted by learning about inner experiences. The patient who describes uncontrollable feelings of anger is at greater risk of behaving violently than one who does not.

In summary, the fact that mental disorders are defined in terms of behavior and experience requires the psychiatrist both to become more thorough and more skillful in using traditional medical methods of evaluation and to develop new skills that are unlikely to be learned in the process of traditional medical education. The psychiatrist must be skilled in:

1. Helping patients and others accurately describe behavior.
2. Observing behavior as a participant.
3. Taking an extensive history that focuses on past behavior and experience.

4. Helping patients communicate inner experience.
5. Detecting inaccurate communication.
6. Testing for aberrations of perception, thought, and feeling.
7. Determining how behavioral and experiential difficulties may be related.

The manner in which these skills can be learned and applied to the process of evaluation will be discussed in subsequent chapters.

HOW DOES THE MANNER IN WHICH MENTAL ILLNESSES ARE INFLUENCED BY THE ENVIRONMENT AFFECT THE PROCESS OF PSYCHIATRIC EVALUATION?

One reason why mental illnesses are so complicated, so protean in manifestation, and so interesting is that the phenomena which define them—disturbances in behavior and experience—are powerfully influenced by the environment. Physical illnesses are also responsive to the environment, but they are influenced by environmental variables in a more subtle manner and, as a rule, only over prolonged periods of time. The signs and symptoms of mental disorders are characterized by dramatic short-term responsivity to environmental events.

Psychiatric symptoms are peculiarly context-dependent. They can change from hour to hour and even from minute to minute depending on the nature of the environment. Even severely disturbed psychiatric patients whose symptoms appear to have powerful biological determinants may function normally under certain environmental conditions. Most experienced clinicians have observed situations in which extremely regressed psychotic patients have responded to emergencies such as a physical illness or a natural disaster with highly adaptive behavior.

As a resident in psychiatry I had the opportunity to observe the response of an entire ward of chronically psychotic patients to the threat of an impending tornado. Some of these patients were so severely disabled that they often had to be fed or bathed by others. Yet, during a tornado drill, under the realistic threat of death or injury, the entire group behaved impeccably in following directions for self-protection. One patient who had not uttered an intelligible sentence in years was able to provide very coherent instructions to his fellow patients. When the threat of danger ended, he returned to speaking gibberish.

Less drastic changes in the environment can also modify psychotic behavior. There are psychiatric units where patients are given privileges only if they present tokens. These tokens, in turn, can be earned only by behaving in a nonpsychotic manner (this is a so-called token economy).

We know that, under such conditions, the more gross manifestations of the psychotic behavior often disappear. Other psychiatric syndromes such as anorexia nervosa are effectively treated by creating hospital environments in which patients receive reinforcement only if they gain weight. Psychiatrists' awareness of the importance of milieu factors has led to the design of hospital environments that help the patient to behave in an adaptive manner. Here, the environment (or the hospital milieu) becomes a major vector in treatment.

Environmental change may also have the dramatic, short-term effect of worsening psychiatric symptomatology. Psychotic patients, particularly those who have organic impairments, are greatly disturbed by even minor shifts in the physical environment. All psychiatric patients may be profoundly disturbed by environmental events outside their control that involve loss or that put demands on them that they cannot meet.

Even the relationship with the physician can be viewed as an environmental variable that will influence the course of the patient's illness. This is apparent in both the short and the long run.

Examiners for the American Board of Psychiatry and Neurology often have the opportunity to observe two or three psychiatrists interviewing the same patient for the same purpose on the same day. There is usually a very significant variation in the content of these interviews. What happens is that each physician imposes his or her unique environment upon the patient and the patient responds to each environment differently. A similar phenomenon can be observed at teaching conferences when the patient is interviewed by both a skilled and an unskilled clinician. The unskilled clinician may create an interviewing environment in which the patient will become more symptomatic. When the skilled interviewer takes over, the severely disturbed patient may become much more comfortable and may begin to look relatively normal.

The long-term relationship with the physician creates an environment in which many new forms of learning can take place. In and of itself, this relationship often provides enough support so that the patient can behave more adaptively and can experience less suffering. All psychotherapeutic relationships can be conceptualized as efforts to help the patient by creating a new environment in which new adaptive behaviors can be learned and older maladaptive behaviors unlearned.

Because the nature of psychiatric symptomatology is so powerfully shaped by the environment, the psychiatric physician must pay very close attention to the context in which symptomatology occurs. The focus here is usually on levels of stress in current and past environments that are believed to have precipitated new symptomatology or to have exacerbated preexisting symptomatology. One of the most important environments to be assessed here is the one created by the patient's family. The clinician who is aware of family or other environmental stressors is in a better position to try to modify them. The psychiatrist must also be concerned with what happens in the patient's environment once the symptoms of a mental disorder appear. Psychiatric symptomatology generally elicits new responses from the surround (in the form of stress or reinforcement) that may sustain symptoms or make them worse. These environmental responses can also be modified in a manner that helps to diminish the severity of the symptomatology. An analysis of the environment in which symptoms develop and are sustained is not usually viewed as an essential aspect of nonpsychiatric evaluation (even though it probably should be). In psychiatry, an analysis of the influence of the environment is indispensable.

The environment also exerts a long-term influence on behavior and experience. From birth onward, the patient is exposed to a unique social milieu. In the process of developing within this milieu, one may learn patterns of behavior and experience that are maladaptive, or one may fail to learn responses that may be necessary for coping. The nature of the patient's social learning can be a cause of symptomatology or can favor the development of personality traits that complicate symptomatology. Understanding the patient's past learning often allows the physician to provide psychological interventions that help the patient to learn more adaptive responses and to unlearn maladaptive ones.

The psychiatrist learns about how the patient has been influenced by past environments by taking an extensive past history. Such a review is usually much more detailed than is customary in other aspects of medical practice. Every person enters the world with a unique set of potentialities, which are either expressed or inhibited by the manner in which he or she interacts with a unique environment. Properly elicited, the past history is always rich and interesting. It is truly the story of the patient's life and should be pursued in as much depth as time allows. Statements such as "the past history is negative" or the "psychosocial history is unremarkable" are logically incorrect in any medical approach to the patient, but they are especially inappropriate in psychiatric practice.

In summary, the fact that mental disorders are powerfully influenced by the environment requires the psychiatrist to take a much more detailed history than is customary in traditional medicine. This history must focus on the patient's learning experiences in past environments, on the nature of the environment in which the symptoms developed, and on the environmental response to the patient's symptoms. The physician must also consider how current environmental variables, including the physician's own interaction with the patient, will influence the patient's symptomatology.

HOW ARE MENTAL ILLNESSES INFLUENCED BY THOUGHT PROCESSES AND WHAT IS THE SIGNIFICANCE OF THIS INFLUENCE FOR PSYCHIATRIC EVALUATION?

All patients think about their symptoms, but the content of that thought has little immediate impact on most physical symptoms. The patient's thoughts (which are on aspect of her or his experience) do, however, exert a powerful and direct influence on his or her behavior and emotional state (another aspect of the patient's experience). There is now ample evidence from the fields of cognitive therapy and attribution theory that the manner in which individuals think about and explain their environment, their behavior, and their feelings influences how they behave and how they feel. Often, the influence of thinking on symptomatology is readily apparent. Patients who repeatedly view the environment as unfriendly, when in reality it is not, behave inappropriately. Patients who think of themselves as helpless, unloved, or unlovable create or escalate feelings of anxiety and sadness in themselves. Often, the clinician can predict how the patient will behave or can infer a great deal about what the patient may feel, by knowing what the patient is thinking.

Psychiatric evaluation requires meticulous attention to the content of the patient's thoughts. Physicians must first of all be concerned with the presence of irrational thoughts (which may themselves be symptoms) and how they influence the patient's behavior and feeling. They must also be concerned with the patient's motivations and how these are related to the patient's behavior. Finally, they must determine if there are patterns of thinking that are regularly associated with the patient's symptomatology. Some of the patterns are manifestations of personality traits.

HOW ARE MENTAL ILLNESSES INFLUENCED BY PERSONALITY TRAITS, AND WHAT IS THE SIGNIFICANCE OF THIS INFLUENCE FOR PSYCHIATRIC EVALUATION?

In the course of interacting with the environment over time, patients begin to develop consistent and predictable patterns of behaving and experiencing. The manner in which patients perceive, think about, or relate to themselves or to others is of particular interest to psychiatrists. When such behaviors and experiences take on consistent patterns and become pervasive or enduring, we view these patterns as personality traits. When such traits are clearly maladaptive and when they contribute to the patient's distress or disability, we view them as disorders of personality. In standard nomenclature (DSM-III-R), a personality disorder can be the primary or Axis I diagnosis; it is often a secondary or Axis II diagnosis. Whether or not a formal personality diagnosis is actually made, all psychiatric patients do have personality traits that influence the manner in which they deal with any mental illness they may develop.

Physical illnesses are also influenced by personality traits. Indeed, much of the focus of preventive medicine these days is on efforts to change the lifestyle of patients, which is largely a manifestation of their personality traits, in the hopes that such a change will reduce the risk of certain physical illnesses or will help them cope with illnesses that already exist. In nonpsychiatric medicine, however, the influence of personality on symptomatology is chronic and insidious. In psychiatric medicine, this influence is more apparent and may be immediate as well as long-standing.

Personality variables exert a direct influence on how an individual responds to stressful events. Such elements of personality may be critical in determining whether patients' coping mechanisms will be sufficient or insufficient to allow them to avoid symptomatology. Patients described as having narcissistic personality traits, for example, and who constantly seek the approval of others may predictably react to a loss of reinforcement by becoming depressed. Patients with antisocial personality traits are likely to respond to stressful circumstances with abrasive interpersonal behavior such as exploitation of others, lying, or aggressiveness. Patients with paranoid traits may respond to a minor social slight with massive anger.

Knowledge of personality traits also helps the psychiatrist predict how patients are likely to respond to specific psychiatric disabilities. Highly compulsive patients, for example, often cope more successfully with organic brain impairments than those who lack this trait. A patient with antisocial personality traits who develops schizophrenia will usually pose difficult problems with aggression. A patient with histrionic personality traits who becomes depressed may show unpredictable mood swings as the illness develops.

Personality traits also influence responses to treatment. Highly dependent patients may do better with a very structured treatment approach. Paranoid patients may not be willing to comply with some treatment approaches, whereas compulsive patients may be highly compliant. Antisocial patients may lack the motivation to participate in therapeutic enterprises unless they are under duress.

In summary, the clinician's task in evaluating personality traits is threefold: first, to try to describe those personality traits that are present; second, to seek to determine which of these traits are maladaptive; and third, to attempt to ascertain how these traits influence the patient's response to any symptoms of mental disorders that may be present.

Evaluations of personality are made by obtaining a history of the patient's past patterns of perceiving, thinking about, and relating to himself or herself and others. The maladaptive aspects of such traits can be inferred by inquiring into how patients have responded to a variety of past experiences and by noting when these responses have not served them well. Consequently, the physician notes whether any maladaptive patterns are detectable or expressed during the interview. In determining the impact of personality traits on symptoms, the clinician must also explore the manner in which patients perceive, think about, and deal with their disorder. This is a complex aspect of assessment that may require a great deal of inference.

The process of personality assessment is not given as great a priority as it deserves in most forms of medical evaluation. Some medical clinics obtain personality profiles on all patients by using tests such as the Minnesota Multiphasic Personality Inventory (MMPI). The actual evaluation of personality and its impact on illness, however, may not be done by the physician. Even in psychiatry, personality traits may not be routinely assessed as part of the mental status examination. Nor are such traits always described in the history. Among the more psycho-dynamic psychiatrists, considerable emphasis is placed on personality diagnosis. Such an assessment may be described as an evaluation of ego functioning. Neurobiologically oriented psychiatrists are less concerned with how personality traits influence current functioning and tend to make personality diagnoses primarily on the basis of past history.

The approach here is that personality assessment is a critical part of any psychiatric evaluation and can best be accomplished through a combination of history taking and observation of current mental functioning. The aspect of the psychiatric evaluation that deals with personality evaluation should include an assessment of how patients perceive and think about themselves (including self-concept, aspirations, self-esteem, and levels of guilt and self-criticism); how patients think about and relate to other people, to their work, to recreation, and to their illnesses; and how they deal with religious and existential issues. Whether these assessments are best viewed as part of the classical mental status examination or as a separate category of current mental functioning is unimportant. The only critical issue is that these assessments be made.

WHAT ARE SOME OF THE LIMITATIONS OF DIAGNOSIS IN PSYCHIATRY AND HOW DO THEY INFLUENCE EVALUATION?

For the beginning psychiatrist, it is a most frustrating experience to make an accurate diagnosis and then to discover that this exercise is not as helpful in treating or managing the patient as it is in other aspects of medicine. Psychiatric diagnoses do not, in themselves, provide specific guidelines for treatment. This is true because most mental disorders are classified descriptively (on the basis of behavior and experience) rather than etiologically (on the basis of cause). Some medical disorders are, of course, also classified solely on the basis of signs or symptoms. The number of such categories, however, is rapidly diminishing as more is learned about their etiologies. With certain exceptions, such as the organic brain disorders and adjustment reactions, the causes of mental disorders are disputed or unknown. As a result, the best we can do is classify them on the basis of descriptions of clinical features that over time have been observed to be associated with particular outcomes.

The descriptive approach is an essential beginning to the process of diagnosis and treatment. It allows for the prediction of outcome or prognosis. Once the prognosis is known, it is possible to test the efficacy of a variety of interventions that may modify it. A descriptive diagnosis may also provide limited guidelines for treatment. The combined clinical experience of many psychiatrists and other mental health professionals has taught us that certain treatments are likely to be effective for certain diagnostic categories. When we know that something works on the basis of experience, our use of that treatment is described as empirical. Treatment based on empiricism is important in all branches of medicine. There are substantial limits, however, to such an approach, and these limits are very apparent in psychiatry. With the exception of a few disorders, such as bipolar affective disorder or adult adjustment disorder, there is substantial disagreement in psychiatry on which treatments or combinations of treatments are, empirically, most effective in treating specific psychiatric disorders.

All scholarly texts, including the DSM-III-R, fully acknowledge that the process of treatment planning involves much more than just making a diagnosis. For the purposes of treatment, psychiatric evaluation must go beyond diagnosis and is actually based on the clinician's assessment of a wide variety of qualities or variables that describe the individual patient. These include such elements as the patient's physical status, medical history, age, sex, education, family situation, intelligence, legal status, personality traits, occupational status, psychological mindedness, current levels of stress, previous treatment, and previous patterns of achievement and motivation. These variables are assessed during the process of history taking, mental status evaluation, and physical and laboratory examination. They are relevant to treatment planning in two ways. First, some variables, such as age, race, sex, or response to previous treatment, may lead the clinician to make modifications of treatment based on empiricism or experience. Second, an evaluation of patient-related variables may help the clinician to formulate various models of etiology or causation. Even though the clinician may not be certain about the etiology of mental disorders, the model one constructs about what is causing the symptoms in a particular case usually serves as a major guide to treatment.

The need to develop information about patient variables that may be related to etiology once again confronts the psychiatric clinician with the imperative of taking a more extensive history than that required in nonpsychiatric medicine.

IF DIAGNOSIS IS NOT ENOUGH, WHAT CONCEPTUAL FRAMEWORK CAN THE PHYSICIAN USE IN EVALUATING PSYCHIATRIC PATIENTS FOR THE PURPOSE OF TREATMENT?

The major advances in modern medicine have been created by expanding the physician's knowledge of etiology. As the pathophysiology of a disease is understood, the clinician develops a clear idea of what can be done to modify it and where to look to discover new forms of intervention. The value of the expanding knowledge of etiology has been dramatically apparent in the history of psychiatry. Early in this century, psychiatrists learned that symptoms very similar to those of schizophrenia were, in some cases, actually caused by syphilis or pellagra. That knowledge enabled clinicians to use the available treatment for these diseases and to eradicate most of their psychiatric manifestations in modern society. More recently, psychiatrists have learned that some patients who fit most of the diagnostic criteria for major depression have hypothyroidism and that they may be relieved of troubling emotional symptoms by the treatment of this disorder.

As the clinician's understanding of the causation, particularly the biological causation, of mental illness expands, the psychiatric diagnostic system will increasingly be based on etiology and will therefore be much more relevant to treatment. The current understanding of the etiology of mental disorders, however, lags behind the knowledge of the etiology of most other medical disorders. One way of making this point is to consider the names we give to diseases, and what those names symbolize in various branches of medicine. Diagnostic terms such as *myocardial infarction, pulmonary embolism,* or *pneumococcal pneumonia* refer to etiological processes. Other terms, such as *lupus erythematosis* or *multiple sclerosis,* are now associated with a relatively comprehensive understanding of the pathophysiological processes that are producing symptoms. We cannot say the same for diagnosis such as schizophrenia, anxiety disorders, personality disorders, or somatoform disorders. These remain descriptive diagnoses, although there is a growing, but still limited, consensus among behavioral scientists about their causation.

Ultimately, physicians must go beyond empiricism and choose most interventions on the basis of the knowledge or theories of causation. The problem for psychiatrists is that they are provided with many theories of etiology, supported by varying degrees of scientific validation. This situation leaves them with two alternatives. They can grasp onto a single etiological perspective, such as the biological, the behavioral, or the psychodynamic, and base the majority of their interventions on that theoretical framework. Or they can consider a variety of perspectives and provide several forms of treatment based on differing views of causation. The latter approach can be undertaken in a limited or a comprehensive manner. If limited, clinicians may simply acknowledge that more than one explanatory system provides clues to treating the patient's illness and try to determine whether a particular system may be relevant in a given case. The treatment will be more varied than it is when clinicians use only one etiological perspective, and it may indeed take on a "shotgun" quality. If clinicians adopt a more comprehensive approach, which, of course, is recommended here, they need a conceptual framework for considering the relevance of all reasonable hypotheses.

One model for planning treatment is based on the observation that psychiatric symptomatology can be understood as a product of the interaction of three main classes of factors, namely, psychological, biological, and social. The key to conceptualizing this approach to treatment is routinely to consider *all* causative factors and their interactions. Some factors, particularly those that are biological, may at times be more powerful causative agents than others. But other important elements of causation must also be considered. Even for the patient with an organic brain disorder, who has an observable biological deficit, the significant behavior and experiences (or symptomatology) cannot be understood unless a great deal is known about the patient's past learning, personality development, and present and past environmental experience.

A multidimensional approach to causation allows for a broad approach to treatment. Patients can be concurrently treated with several interventions that modify suspected etiological processes. Biological intervention can be provided to ameliorate biochemical malfunctions. New learning experiences can be created to supplement or change maladaptive past learning. Efforts can be made to create new environments for patients that are free of the interpersonal and social stresses that may have played a role in the development of their illnesses.

This method of treatment planning is facilitated when the physician considers etiology in terms of classes of hypotheses of causation. During the process of history taking and mental status examination, it is useful for the clinician to consider the following categories of hypotheses:

1. *Biological hypotheses.* Here, the clinician considers the possibility

that the patient's mental disorder has genetic or acquired biological determinants. Any clinical or laboratory evidence that suggests a structural or pathophysiological dysfunction is noted. The manner in which the biological characteristics may have influenced the patient's social learning is explored. The patient's current physical status is studied for the way in which various deficits may contribute to psychopathology.

Biological hypotheses suggest the need for biological interventions in the form of pharmacotherapy, electroconvulsive therapy, or the treatment of underlying physical conditions.

2. *Learning hypotheses*. Here, the clinician considers the nature of the patient's learning experiences by focusing on the patient's unique biological characteristics, and how these have influenced and have been influenced by the various environments in which the patient has interacted up to the present. The clinician investigates how maladaptive past learning leads to impairments in the patient's capacity to cope with the current environment. This kind of evaluation is guided by two types of questions: What has the patient learned in the past that contributes to symptoms in the present? And what has the patient failed to learn in the past, which if acquired, might have prevented or alleviated the symptoms in the present? Learning hypotheses suggest a need for behavioral interventions in which maladaptive responses are unlearned, and in which more adaptive responses are learned. This aspect of behavior modification is also an integral part of all psychotherapy.

3. *Informational hypotheses*. Here, the clinician considers four classes of hypotheses that explain symptomatic behavior as related to informational deficits. These hypotheses can be phrased in terms of the following questions:

   a. What information does the patient lack about how he or she influences the environment (as a rule, *environment*, in this context, means "other people")? One who does not know how he or she comes across to others cannot modify maladaptive behavior such as seductiveness or aggressiveness.
   b. What information does the patient lack about how the environment (usually other people) influences him or her? One who does not know how others affect him or her cannot deal with them in an adaptive manner.
   c. What information does the patient lack about how past experience influences current behavior? One who does not know how current behavior is shaped by past experience has an imprecise view of what behavior or feelings are important to change.
   d. What information does the patient lack about what others (the environment) expect of him or her? The patient cannot behave in a socially adaptive manner unless he or she knows what the environment demands.

Answers to these four questions suggest the use of interventions that expand the patient's information, usually through individual, group, or family psychotherapy. Most psychotherapy is based on both informational and learning hypotheses. Psychodynamic or psychoanalytic psychotherapy emphasizes expanding information about how the past influences the present, how the unconscious influences the conscious, and how one dimension of the mind may influence another (how the superego affects the ego).

4. *Environmental hypotheses*. Here, the physician considers how current stresses influence the patient's symptomatology. The therapist also notes how current patterns of reinforcement in the environment may perpetuate symptomatology or may prevent the learning of more adaptive responses. Environmental hypotheses suggest the use of interventions that change the environment (e.g., family therapy, case management techniques, or behavior modification).

HOW DOES THE ISSUE OF THE PATIENT'S CAPACITIES INFLUENCE PSYCHIATRIC EVALUATION?

All physicians must, at times, evaluate their patients' capacities to perform various tasks. The nonpsychiatric physician is usually concerned with patients' physical capacities and, most commonly, with the extent to which they can exert themselves at various tasks without making their condition worse. In making this kind of assessment, the doctor considers the manner in which anatomical and physiological deficiencies influence the patient's functional capacities. This assessment may have legal implications when the patient is seeking disability compensation, or it may be purely a matter of clinical management when the patient must be advised whether to pursue ordinary activities or to stay home and rest in bed.

The psychiatrist has the much broader task of assessing not only how mental impairments influence patients' capacity to perform occupational tasks, but also how they influence patients' capacity to behave in a socially acceptable manner and to make adaptive choices. In the clinical context, the psychiatrist is routinely asked to make decisions about whether it is helpful for patients to continue to tend to their daily tasks or should be assigned less strenuous tasks that may have therapeutic value. The psychiatrist must also make decisions about patients' capacity to behave rationally in various social settings. If patients are judged to lack such capacity, they are likely to be treated in a more controlled environment. The psychiatrist may also be asked whether patients have the capacity to choose to continue at certain tasks or to abstain from them, to seek hospital care voluntarily, to manage their own affairs, or to cooperate with the treatment plan by submitting to procedures or taking medications. Many of these assessments have legal implications and are carefully monitored by the courts.

Unless the physician develops an interest in forensic medicine, he or she is unlikely to receive much training in evaluating capacities. The requisite skills are almost never considered in basic medical texts. Yet, the problem of relating the patients' psychological impairments to their functional capacity to make choices and perform tasks is a very practical one. It is an important part of medical practice and an indispensable part of psychiatric practice from the first day of residency training. In dealing with inpatients, the psychiatrist must make daily judgments of their capacities to benefit from a variety of interpersonal, recreational, and occupational experiences. With voluntary patients, such assessments lead to the physician's prescribing activities that the patient agrees to carry out. Often, however, it is impossible to prescribe therapeutic activity until patients have been adjudicated to be so lacking the *capacity* to choose treatment that others must make treatment decisions for them. This means that the beginning psychiatrist must also participate in civil commitment proceedings in which he or she must present an opinion on the patient's capacities to refrain from antisocial or self-injurious conduct. In many jurisdictions, the first-year resident must also assist the courts in determining whether the patient possesses or lacks the capacity to refuse treatment.

The psychiatrist's obligation to evaluate a variety of behavioral, perceptual, cognitive, and emotional capacities requires him or her to pay more attention to how the patient has functioned in the past. It is important to know how patients have performed various functions when free of impairment and how past impairments have influenced their current functional capacities. Similar considerations apply to the quality of the patient's choices. The psychiatrist must also make estimates of how various current impairments may influence the patient's current and future functioning. Usually, these estimates require a detailed evaluation of experiential variables, particularly of the patient's capacities to perceive and think rationally.

Because the subject of the assessment of capacity is so important and has received so little attention in most psychiatric texts, this issue will be explored in a brief chapter at the end of this book.

HOW DOES THE ISSUE OF SOCIAL CONTROL INFLUENCE PSYCHIATRIC EVALUATION?

In addition to being influenced by the environment, mental disorders also have an impact on the environment. Here, the behavioral manifestations of mental illness are most important. Some of the associated behavior, such as aggressiveness, dependency, or failure to adhere to social norms, may have a direct and negative impact on the community. Deviant conduct is usually frightening to many in society, especially when it seems to be unreasonable. The common assumption that the mentally ill cannot exercise the same control over their behavior as do normal people adds to the community's concern that the mentally ill are dangerous. When dangerousness is suspected, the community may wish to restrict the freedom of such patients by hospitalizing them. The community may also be concerned that the mentally ill will do great harm if put in positions of responsibility in society, particularly positions that involve public safety. A high level of concern is expressed when there is even a remote possibility that police officers, government officials, airplane pilots, physicians, or attorneys may be mentally ill.

Society's concerns that the mentally ill will exert a disruptive or harmful effect on the social order are often realistic. This concern, in turn, leads to efforts to control some aspects of the behavior of such patients by restricting their freedom or their access to positions of responsibility. In exerting this form of social control, society generally calls on the evaluative skills of psychiatrists. These clinicians are asked to become involved in the process of civil commitment, to help determine which patients should be deprived of freedom, for what length of time, and in what setting. Psychiatrists are also asked which patients should be denied or granted social benefits such as disability income, and which patients should be denied or granted access to certain professional statuses or jobs. (As noted in the previous section, in these evaluative roles the psychiatrist is trying to determine how mental illness influences various aspects of the patient's capacities.) The psychiatrist may not make the final decision about what will happen to the patient, but his or her recommendations invariably influence that outcome.

When the psychiatrist assists society in making decisions that may have major social consequences for patients, it is often the case that patients do not perceive the psychiatrist's recommendations as helpful to them. These perceptions may be accurate. Interventions designed to control a patient's behavior may not always have a salutary influence on the patient's experience of well-being. Members of the patient's community may be pleased when the patient is restricted, but the patient may feel worse.

When psychiatrists evaluate a patient for the purpose of treatment, their primary allegiance is to the patient. They may not harm the patient except through negligence. When psychiatrists evaluate the patient for commitment, employment, or some other legal determination, however, even when psychiatrists do their job well, the patient remains at risk of perceived or actual harm. In this situation, it may be fairly said that psychiatrists often have greater allegiance to the social agency that employs them than to the patient.

The assumption of a role in which allegiance to an agency may be greater than to the patient is not unique to psychiatric physicians. When doctors of any specialty evaluate patients for potential employability, insurability, or disability, they are agency-employed, and their recommendations may not be welcomed by their patients. All physicians also become agents of social control when they follow the requirements of law and report gunshot wounds, certain communicable diseases, and suspected cases of child abuse. The difference in psychiatry is the greater frequency with which psychiatrists are agency- rather than patient-employed, and the extent to which psychiatrists must participate in social control functions. A sizable proportion of psychiatric practice, *and particularly that which the beginning resident encounters*, involves evaluating patients at the request of agencies rather than at the request of patients themselves.

Throughout the history of psychiatry, the problem of how to evaluate a patient who does not voluntarily seek the psychiatrist's attention, and who in fact may resent it, has been inherent in psychiatric practice. It has major ethical and practical implications that are too often ignored by all mental health professionals. The practical aspects of evaluating a patient for an agency will be discussed in other chapters. Here, some of the ethical issues that make psychiatric evaluation somewhat different from the evaluation of other medical conditions are briefly noted.

Accurate psychiatric evaluation usually requires a cooperative patient. In psychiatry, cooperation means more than passive participation by answering questions or submitting to a physical examination. If they are to be adequately evaluated, psychiatric patients must reveal as much as they can about their past behavior, their thoughts, and their feelings. There are a number of ways of enhancing the patient's cooperativeness. Psychiatrists try to maximize the patient's self-disclosure by the use of techniques such as communicating empathy, asking relevant questions, and selectively reinforcing certain patient responses (these techniques will be described in subsequent sections). All of these methods were developed in order to help patients. A critical conflict arises when the psychiatrist uses tactics designed primarily to help patients in order to garner information that may be used to recommend outcomes that the patients may not welcome.

There are no easy resolutions to the conflicts that arise when the psychiatrist assumes social-control (sometimes called *double-agent*) roles. There is, however, one major guideline that the student can rely on that may make the ethical dilemma somewhat less oppressive. Psychiatric evaluators are under special obligation to make certain that the patient fully understands the purpose of any evaluation. If the psychiatrist's findings can be used to initiate outcomes that the patient may not welcome, the patient must be fully aware of that possibility. Most patients have learned to view doctors as helping persons. It is difficult for them to appreciate that their evaluator may have allegiances to others, and that these obligations may eventually have an adverse influence on them (the patients). The ethical doctrine of *informed consent* does help reduce the possibility of harm to patients. Psychiatric evaluators are obligated to make the possible outcomes of evaluation absolutely clear to patients. The patient must be informed of the doctor's allegiance, the purpose of the evaluation, who will see the doctor's report, and how it may be used to influence decisions about the patient's freedom or privileges.

Lest beginning psychiatrists fear that too much involvement in social control functions will destroy their integrity as physicians, it is useful to consider the reality that social control functions can also be helpful to the patient. In many situations, even though the patient may perceive an outcome of psychiatric evaluation as harmful, there is still a high probability that it will eventually be helpful. In some social control situations, the needs of society and the needs of the individual are congruent. Involuntary commitment does not harm patients, if it ultimately helps to restore their health. Denying a patient access to a socially responsible position is not a harm, if that patient truly lacks the capacity to meet the obligations that are part of that position.

Most of the time the psychiatrist's social control functions help patients or at least do not harm them. Those situations in which psychiatric evaluations lead to outcomes that are not in the patient's ultimate interest are most likely to arise in forensic psychiatry. There, psychiatrist's reports may be used by legal agencies to impose punishment or deny compensation. In such instances, the ethical dilemmas cannot usually be resolved by trying to help the patient and the social agency at the same time. This type of forensic evaluation may be inconsistent with the basic medical ethical principal of *primum non noncere*. Whenever possible, beginning psychiatrists should be shielded from having to participate in forensic evaluations that may have highly aversive consequences for patients.

IS IT REALLY POSSIBLE TO MASTER THE COMPLEXITY OF PSYCHIATRIC EVALUATION, AND IS IT WORTH DOING?

By now, the student should be painfully aware of the reality that psychiatric evaluation is difficult and complex. It is not, however, unlearnable. As students practice the skills involved in a thorough and systematic accumulation of data, and as they reflect about these data in a systematic manner, they will get better and better. It is also true that there are ample rewards for mastering this process. First, in using a systems-oriented or biopsychosocial model, a psychiatrist has the privilege of setting a standard of practice for all other physicians. By dealing with the influence of the critical psychosocial factors, which are so often ignored in other branches of medicine, the psychiatrist can practice the most comprehensive and, ultimately, the most humanistic medicine. Second, learning psychiatric evaluation liberates the clinician to study issues that go beyond biomedical causation. The well-trained psychiatrist is "at work" when he or she is studying neurotransmitters, theology, poverty, or poetry. Finally, the complexity of psychiatric evaluation precludes boredom. Each patient is a unique experience in the psychiatrist's life. The evaluation of psychiatric patients, properly conducted, provides the psychiatrist with unlimited opportunities to learn, to wonder, and to be surprised.

FOR FURTHER READING

Akiskal, H. A. The classification of mental disorders. In *Comprehensive textbook of psychiatry, Vol. 5.* H. I. Kaplan and B. J. Sadock, (Eds.). Williams & Wilkins, Baltimore, 1989.

American Psychiatric Association. *Diagnostic and statistical manual of mental disorders (3rd ed., rev.).* Washington, D.C., 1987.

Dubovsky, S. L. *A concise guide to clinical psychiatry.* American Psychiatric Association Press, Washington, D.C., 1988.

Gill, M., Newman, R., and Redlich, F. *The initial interview in psychiatric practice.* International University Press, New York, 1954.

Halleck, S. L. *Psychiatry and the dilemmas of crime.* Harper, New York, 1967.

Halleck, S. L. *Treatment of emotional disorders.* Aronson Press, New York, 1978.

The Hastings Center. In the service of the state: The psychiatrist as double agent (special supplement), The Hastings Center, Hastings-on-Hudson, 1978.

Karasu, T. B. The psychiatric therapies. *The APA Commission on Psychiatric Therapies*, American Psychiatric Press, Washington, D.C., 1984.

Klerman, G. L. Valliant, G. E., Spitzer, R. C., and Michels, R. A debate on DSM-III. *American Journal of Psychiatry*, 141:539–553, 1984.

MacKinnon, R., and Michels, R. *The psychiatric interview in clinical practice.* W. B. Saunders, Philadelphia, 1971.

Menninger, K. *A manual for psychiatric case study.* Grune & Stratton, New York, 1952.

Reid, W. H., and Wise, M. C. *DSM-III: A training guide.* Brunner/Mazel, New York, 1989.

Schwartz, H. S., and Roth, L. H. Informed consent and competency in psychiatric practice. Chapter 20, *Review of psychiatry*, A. B. Tasman, R. B. Hales, and A. J. Francis (Eds.). American Psychiatric Press, Washington, D.C., 1989.

Skodol, A. E., and Spitzer, R. L. *An annotated bibliography of DSM-III.* American Psychiatric Association Press, 1987.

Spitzer, R. L., Williams, J., and Skodol, A. E. DSM-III: The major achievements and an overview. *American Journal of Psychiatry*, 137:151–164, 1988.

CHAPTER TWO

Obtaining Information from the Patient

Psychiatric evaluation is a process in which the physician seeks to obtain as much relevant information as possible about the patient. This process is, of course, subject to the constraints of time. Even in the most rarefied academic atmosphere, there is rarely sufficient time to do as complete an examination as the clinician might wish. It is helpful for the examiner to begin the interview with some idea of how much time is available, and what specific information will be sought. As a rule, the information garnered in the psychiatric evaluation must also be communicated to other professionals or social agencies. Hence, the physician must also have some idea about how much information will be recorded in the patient's chart.

The first part of this chapter deals with the manner in which the physician can use the available time to collect and record as much relevant information as possible. No matter how much time is available, however, there are always certain factors that may impede or facilitate the process of information gathering. The second part of this chapter is an effort to describe these factors and to help the clinician learn to deal with them in a manner that maximizes the flow of information.

HOW DO PATIENTS COME TO BE
EVALUATED BY THE PSYCHIATRIST?

Psychiatrists treat patients in both the outpatient and the hospital setting. Some outpatients are in urgent need of care and may walk in or may be brought to regular clinics or emergency rooms. Other outpatients, whose distress or disability is not viewed by themselves or their physicians as requiring immediate care, may arrange to be seen on an appointment basis.

Outpatient visits can be either voluntary or involuntary. Many patients actively seek help on their own. Others may experience their visits as coerced, either by family members, by fear of loss of employment, or by threats of possible civil commitment. The degree of voluntariness of help seeking in these situations is quite variable. If the patient is told, "Get a psychiatric evaluation or lose your job," or, "If you don't see the psychiatrist, I'll sign these commitment papers," the patient experiences little or no sense of choice.

Still other patients visit psychiatrists to obtain forensic examinations that may have a bearing on their employability, their quest for worker's compensation, or the outcome of criminal or civil litigation in which they are involved. Depending on whether they view the examining psychiatrist as a potential helper or as an adversary, they will approach the examination with varying degrees of enthusiasm. Finally, patients who are brought to the psychiatrist on petition for civil commitment are there involuntarily and may resist the process of evaluation.

Inpatients on psychiatric wards may be voluntary or involuntary. Psychiatrists also see inpatients on medical-surgical wards when they provide consultation to other doctors. On either a psychiatric or a nonpsychiatric unit, a certain number of patients have urgent medical or psychiatric problems that require immediate attention. Others are medically stabilized, and it is possible to conduct their evaluations on a scheduled basis.

The parameters of the degree of voluntariness, the locus of evaluation (in- or outpatient), and the degree of urgency all have some influence on the manner in which the physician goes about collecting information from the patient. These parameters are considered throughout the text. The issue of urgency has a direct influence on the psychiatrist's approach. Patients seen in the emergency room or a walk-in clinic or inpatients who are in severe psychological or medical distress must be seen immediately. Sometimes, a psychiatrist can schedule these patients, but more frequently, their care requires putting off other appointments or scheduled activities. Both the urgency of the situation and the need of the psychiatrist to get back to other scheduled activities may then require that the initial assessment be brief rather than comprehensive.

WHEN TIME IS AVAILABLE, WHAT GENERAL CATEGORIES OF INFORMATION DOES THE CLINICIAN SEEK?

In this text, the following categories of information will be considered:

1. The reason why the patient has requested or has been sent for evaluation at this particular time. In most branches of medicine, this part of the evaluation is described as the chief complaint. Psychiatric patients, however, may not have a chief complaint or may have great difficulty enunciating it.
2. The events that precede and that may determine why the patient is seeking or has been sent for help. This information is usually referred to as the history of the present illness. It is essentially a chronology of what has happened (or, more precisely, how the patient has interacted with the environment, usually in a maladaptive manner), from the time just preceding the symptoms until the present.
3. The patient's past medical history, including all psychiatric symptoms and previous psychiatric treatment. It is convenient to consider the family health history (i.e., the mental and physical illnesses in the extended family) under this heading.
4. The patient's past history, including childhood development, educational experiences, work and military experience, and patterns of relating to others. The family relationship history may be included here. Some of the most significant past history deals with the manner in which the patient has interacted with parents, siblings, spouse, or children.
5. The patient's current life situation. Here, two factors are evaluated: first, the patient's current environment, with an emphasis on how it contributes to the patient's symptomatology, and second, an effort to describe the predominant personality traits or manner of relating to himself or herself and the world that the patient brings to the present situation. This information should help clarify how the patient's difficulties have developed, and how the patient is coping with them. Information about personality traits it obtained by reviewing the past history and by observing the patient's responses throughout the evaluation.
6. The patient's current mental status. This should include both observation of the patient's appearance and behavior in the interview and assessment of the patient's perception, cognitive abilities, thoughts, and feeling.
7. The patient's current physical condition is revealed by physical examination (including a neurological examination) and routine laboratory studies.

The above categories may provide guidelines for further evaluation procedures such as CT, an electroencephalogram, endocrinological studies, or psychological testing.

HOW DOES THE PSYCHIATRIST COMPROMISE IN EFFORTS
TO OBTAIN INFORMATION WHEN TIME IS LIMITED?

The range of time the psychiatrist may spend in the evaluative process may vary from twenty to thirty minutes in the emergency room to hundreds of hours in highly publicized forensic cases. Most experienced clinicians devote an average of one to two hours to evaluating each patient. Beginning residents in psychiatry may spend five to ten hours on the evaluation process in the inpatient setting and considerably less time in outpatient clinics. In nonemergency situations, the key variables that determines the length of evaluation are the availability of the physician's and the patient's time, the patient's cooperativeness, the physician's belief system about the depth of evaluation that is necessary, institutional regulations, and economic constraints.

Although the variation in time spent on evaluation in psychiatry is in itself an intriguing issue, the focus here is on how the beginning psychiatrist can adjust to varying time limits with the least sacrifice of accuracy. It is generally true that the accuracy of psychiatric evaluation is directly proportional to the amount of time spent in doing it. As the time available for evaluation lessens, and particularly as it becomes reduced to less than two hours, certain comprises have to be made. The clinician needs to determine which information is most essential, and what inquiries can be abbreviated, postponed, or deleted.

If only twenty to thirty minutes are available for evaluation (assuming the patient's vital signs are normal and there are no indications of physical distress), the evaluation should focus on (1) the reasons for the patient's seeking or being sent for evaluation now; (2) a history of current and past medical problems; (3) the severity of the symptoms and the current level of functioning; (4) suicidal or homicidal ideation; and (5) other aspects of the mental status examination. These are the areas which are most likely to provide relevant information about the nature of the patient's disorder, its seriousness, and its possible impact on the environment and the need for urgent intervention.

If the patient is communicating clearly and articulately, the clinician may have the luxury of postponing some aspects of the mental status exam (such as examining cognitive processes) and may focus more intensively on the patient's reasons for seeking help and the history of the present illness.

Most beginning clinicians are pleasantly surprised to discover how much can be learned in thirty minutes. A good evaluator can often learn why the patient has come for help *now*, can take a medical history, can assess current functioning and that of violence, and can do a brief mental status examination while still having time to pursue other information. The extra time can be most expeditiously used to obtain more history of the present illness, and to asses the nature of the patient's support systems; usually, there is even time to obtain brief personal and family history.

Although it is necessary that students learn how to do a brief evaluation, it is even more imperative that they remain constantly aware of the risk that such an evaluation is likely to be inaccurate. Failing to do a physical and neurological examination as soon as possible is especially risky. Most of the time, these examinations should be done immediately, and there only are a few situations that justify postponing them for more than twenty-four hours. Any abbreviation of history taking also compromises accuracy. Failure to focus sufficiently on the history of the present illness and on the past family history can result in insufficient knowledge of factors relevant to the development of symptoms; in particular, some of these factors may be modifiable. It is also true that many aspects of the mental examination, such as how patients are thinking, what they are thinking about, and what their true emotions are at that moment, are best revealed when patients can tell their story leisurely, over a period of hours rather than minutes.

In most situations, the student should consider the abbreviated evaluation a prelude to a more intensive study. Hopefully, many of the inquiries that were left out of the original evaluation can be pursued during the course of treatment in either an inpatient or an outpatient setting.

Finally, as in all other aspects of medicine, the student should be reminded that shortcuts are best taken by experienced clinicians. There is no substitute for the student's practicing comprehensive evaluations dozens of times before beginning to use an abbreviated format. This is one of the more tried-and-true pedagogic techniques used in most aspects of medical training. In the old days (about a decade ago), residents were required to spend at least five to ten hours in the evaluation of at least a few patients before being encouraged to do briefer evaluations. In many of our training programs, this practice is rapidly disappearing; this, in turn, raises serious concerns about the competency of future psychiatric practitioners.

WHAT INFORMATION SHOULD BE
RECORDED IN THE PATIENT'S CHART?

As a rule, the psychiatrist obtains more information about the patient than can conveniently be put in the chart. Nevertheless, there are several reasons for making the evaluative report as comprehensive as possible. From an economic perspective, a comprehensive written report improves the chart, increases the likelihood of meeting the requirements of insurers, and decreases the risk of malpractice. From a clinical standpoint, the properly recorded evaluation is a source of useful information to other physicians and professionals who will work with the patient. It is also a record for the original evaluator, who over time may forget some of this material. In addition, a good chart serves as an important source for future research. Finally, the very process of recording evaluative material helps the clinician think about and conceptualize the case, a process that is especially important for beginners.

At the same time, there are cogent reasons for keeping psychiatric reports as succinct as possible. The psychiatrist's time is limited. Every moment spent writing a report is a moment spent away from patients. Overly lengthy reports may contain many irrelevancies, and other professionals and physicians who interact with the patient may be reluctant to read them.

Psychiatric institutions have differing rules about how the evaluation should be recorded in the patient's chart. There may be variations in the required length of the report and in the order in which different components of the evaluation are described. There is almost always some variation in the extent to which the various components of the evaluation are emphasized. In many hospital units these days, the psychiatrist is required to record only the chief complaint, the history of the present illness, the medical history, the mental status examination, and the physical examination. The past history, the family history, and the descriptions of personality traits are either noted in a perfunctory manner or reported by some other professional, usually a social worker. Other institutions still require the psychiatrist to record a comprehensive history.

Of course, residents or medical students have to adhere to the rules of the institution in which they work, but they should always be aware of what is being compromised if too much material is deleted. If, for example, historical data are described in a separate section by a social worker, the evaluator may not have the opportunity to conceptualize how this material is related to the patient's present difficulty. The reader of the chart will have similar difficulty in linking past events to present symptomatology. If the history of the present illness is overly compressed, the evaluator and the reader may forget or be unaware of many aspects of the patient's situation (such as a family member's response to the patient's symptomatology) that can be easily ameliorated.

Given the limitations of time and institutional regulations, how can the student record the most clinically useful report? The general answer to this question is that it is helpful to include any material that is relevant to treatment. This means that the student should emphasize information that is relevant to biopsychosocial causation, or that is empirically relevant to treatment. Some institutions may emphasize biological and others psychosocial causation. Although students may have to bend to the wishes of the institution, they should strive to adopt as multidimensional a view of causation as their mentors will allow.

Variations in emphasis in clinical reporting may also be related to the different purposes of reporting. If the purpose of the report is primarily to assist in the process of hospital treatment, the psychiatrist will want to emphasize any characteristics of patients that may influence the way in which they relate themselves to other patients or to the staff. This is much less important if the psychiatrist plans to treat a patient in an outpatient setting. If the report is prepared for an agency that needs to know about certain of the patient's capacities, the evaluator must emphasize historical data and aspects of present mental functioning that help describe these capacities.

HOW DOES THE QUALITY OF COMMUNICATION BETWEEN THE DOCTOR AND THE PATIENT INFLUENCE THE ACCURACY OF THE EVALUATIVE PROCESS?

In most medical evaluations, the primary source of information is the patient's communication about his or her past and present behavior and experience. Others' observations about how the patient behaves or has behaved are also important; however, the most critical determinants of accuracy in evaluation are likely to be the patient's own revelation of his or her current symptoms and past history. The problems that medical practitioners have in evaluating small children or patients whose level of consciousness is diminished attest to how much physicians rely on the patient's communication in making accurate diagnoses. In psychiatry, the clinician is even more concerned about the patient's capacity for communication. A noncommunicative patient not only fails to reveal his or her experiences but also deprives the diagnostician of the opportunity to evaluate how the patient goes about the process of communicating.

Occasionally, psychiatric patients may be unable or unwilling to communicate at all. Mutism may be encountered in patients with severe organic impairment, in catatonia, in severe depression, in some dissociative states, in disturbed children, and in a variety of situations (often related to forensic evaluation) in which the patient believes that any communication with the therapist is risky. Complete silence as a response to any of these disorders or situations, however, is rare. What is more common in psychiatric patients is insufficient or inadequate communication. Nonpsychiatric patients generally have the ability and the motivation to present rather complete descriptions of their symptoms and history. Psychiatric patients may lack the capacity or the will to make a full disclosure of their difficulties. It is also rare for non-psychiatric patients to present inaccurate or distorted information. Psychiatric patients, however, often present distorted versions of their experiences. They are more likely than other patients to communicate inaccurately. They are also more likely to resist "playing by the rules" that govern most aspects of doctor–patient interaction and medical evaluation. Therefore, the psychiatric clinician who strives for accuracy must have some skills in determining when communication is insufficient or inaccurate, must understand some of the reasons why the patient is not communicating clearly, and must develop techniques of interviewing that maximize the flow of accurate information.

HOW DOES THE PSYCHIATRIST DETERMINE WHEN THE PATIENT IS WITHHOLDING INFORMATION OR IS PRESENTING INACCURATE INFORMATION?

Sometimes, the psychiatrist has access to relatively accurate information about the patient from previous records or from reports made by the patient's friends or relatives. If this is the case, it is not too hard to determine when the patient is leaving out significant information or to suspect that the information may be inaccurate. Most of the time, however, clinicians suspect incomplete or inaccurate communication on the basis of wisdom gained through their own life experiences and their experience in evaluating and treating a great many patients. As psychiatrists interview more patients, they expand their awareness of what kind of information is usually provided in the course of evaluation. *Experienced interviewers then become suspicious when that information is not forthcoming.* In the process of treating single patients over time, the psychiatrist also learns that many patients' initial communications were insufficient or inaccurate and may also come to understand why a patient was not more self-disclosing or accurate. Knowledge of what was truly happening in the lives of patients who had complaints similar to that of the patient currently in evaluation alerts the psychiatrist to an awareness of gaps and distortions in the current patient's presentation.

In addition to relying on clinical experience, there are also certain cues that alert the clinician to be concerned about the sufficiency or accuracy of communication. Some of the more obvious ones follow:

1. The patient may answer questions only briefly even when invited or urged to expand on these answers.

2. The patient may not provide details about symptomatology or history even when requested to do so, giving statements of ignorance or amnesia, such as "I don't know" or "I don't remember," changing the subject, or changing his or her attitudes toward the interviewer (usually

in the direction of becoming more angry). All of these responses may be preceded by nonverbal cues that suggest that the patient is anxious, embarrassed, or angered by the doctor's questions.

3. The patient may at various times present contradictory information. During one part of the interview, a patient may say, "I get so depressed that at times I want to end my life," and later the patient may insist, "My symptoms aren't so bad; my family just worries too much."

4. The patient may try to take control of the interview by insisting on limiting disclosures only to subjects of his or her choosing.

5. The patient's communications may not always be logically responsive to the clinician's inquiries or may not be understandable. Here, it is usually apparent that the patient is having trouble either in understanding the examiner or in organizing and communicating his or her own thinking. Sometimes, patients are only occasionally illogical, tangential, or irrelevant; once this is noted, one should question the accuracy of the information provided even when they appear to communicate in a more understandable manner.

6. The patient may be obviously exaggerating. Sometimes, patients exaggerate symptoms ("When I have these headaches I go blind for hours at a time"; "The pain is so bad that I haven't been able to sleep, eat, or sit down for four days"). Sometimes, patients exaggerate their personal abilities or their assets. A frail, elderly patient may emphasize sexual or athletic prowess; an obviously destitute patient may brag about his wealth.

7. Patients may deny the existence of experiences or events that would be easily inferred from their behavior or their current life situation. The patient who breaks out in tears and insists that he or she is feeling fine is an obvious example. Or a patient who is brought in by the police in restraints and insists that he or she was just walking down the street peacefully when picked up by the police and brought to the hospital is another.

8. The patient may respond positively an unusual number of times to questions such as, "Do you have crying spells?" or "Have you ever been in trouble with the law?" Patients who acknowledge or describe symptomatology or adverse experiences too readily may be very poor reporters of events and experiences. Their willingness to own problems that do not exist makes it difficult for the clinician to evaluate the severity of problems that do exist.

9. The patient may repeatedly deny commonplace and universal experience. The patient who responds to a question such as "Do you ever feel angry?" with an unmitigated negative response is either a poor observer of his or her own feelings or is communicating dishonestly.

10. Patients may paint an idyllic picture of their past life and current situation. While this kind of reporting may be accurate in some in-

stances, it is not likely to reflect the reality experienced by most psychiatric patients nor, for that matter, by most people.

11. The patient may simply state that there are some things that he or she is unwilling or unable to discuss. This tells the clinician that there will be substantial gaps in the patient's communication.

WHY DO PATIENTS WITHHOLD INFORMATION?

There are many possible explanations for the patient's withholding information. Sometimes, the patient lacks the cognitive or expressive capacities to communicate essential data to the evaluator. This is true of many patients with organic brain disorders, particularly patients with cortical dysfunctions that produce impairments in the use of language. It may also be true of some patients with dissociative disorders, who experience difficulty in recalling important personal events. Other patients perceive the interview situation as so stressful as to engender a severe degree of anxiety; this, in turn, diminishes their capacity to think and communicate clearly. Patients who are too anxious may forget essential facts or may have great difficulty in presenting a coherent picture of their situation.

Sometimes, psychiatric patients have the capacity to communicate essential data but choose to withhold it intentionally. It may seem paradoxical that a person seeking help would be less than fully candid with the person who is supposed to provide that help; nonetheless, this is often the case. To be sure, the phenomenon of intentional withholding of information occurs in all branches of medicine; in psychiatry, however, it is encountered routinely. Even the most cooperative patient may be unwilling to divulge critical information in the early stages of evaluation.

One of the main reasons that psychiatric patients deliberately withhold information is to avoid humiliation. They feel that they will be overwhelmingly embarrassed by what they reveal. Patients may believe that some of the information they are asked to provide to the physician will reveal their previously hidden shortcomings, especially their failure to have behaved in accordance with their ethical standards or principles. The revelation of one's personal inadequacies, particularly to a stranger, is often accompanied by the distinctly unpleasant emotional state of shame. Most patients with psychiatric disorders do feel a great deal of shame; this may attach to past events, or it may be connected to present thoughts and feelings (perhaps those associated with their illness). In the course of evaluation, as patients are asked about their symptomatology and their history, they are concerned that they will be painfully reminded of their shortcomings. One way in which they can avoid this pain is simply to forgo talking about material that elicits feelings of shame.

Patients may be particularly reluctant to reveal the severity of their problems in thinking or feeling. A certain amount of shame may be involved here, but there is an additional element of fear. Patients who are having difficulty remembering or organizing their thoughts, or who are experiencing bizarre or intrusive thoughts, may fear impending destruction of their sense of "being" or humanness. These fears may be internally expressed in terms of "I'm losing my mind." The fear of loss of the capacity to think clearly is so powerful that patients ordinarily try to hide such a perceived shortcoming from both themselves and others. Even if they acknowledge a problem to themselves, they may be careful to avoid revealing their thoughts to the physician, who has the power to pronounce them "crazy" or to restrict their freedom.

Information regarding the intensity or the perceived deviancy of feelings may be withheld for similar reasons. Patients are often fearful of acknowledging the depth of their anxiety or depression to themselves or to their physician. In addition to being ashamed of what they may perceive as inappropriate feelings (such as anger or sexual desire), such patients may fear that the presence of these feelings threatens their sense of self-control. They may also fear that acknowledgment of such feelings to others will cause others to fear them and to seek to have them hospitalized involuntarily. For all of the above reasons, it is not uncommon for patients who actually have severe mental disorders to present themselves as being asymptomatic or only mildly troubled and perplexed about why they were sent to the psychiatrist in the first place.

Another factor that may impede communication is the patient's perception of the evaluator. Very sick patients sometimes misperceive the therapist as someone who may deliberately wish to hurt them. Less disturbed patients may believe that the evaluator is uninterested in their problems, or that, if the clinician is interested, he or she is either unwilling or unable to help them.

Most people do not view psychiatrists as favorably as they do other physicians. It is useful for the beginning psychiatrist to be aware of this reality. There is great skepticism in our society about the psychiatrist's power to heal. At the same time, there is great concern about the psychiatrist's perceived power to deprive people of liberty. Many patients also perceive psychiatrists as "shrinks," who will tell them that their symptoms are "all in their head" or "just psychological." Such statements are feared by patients because they imply that the patient's symptoms are willfully created, and that they will be subjected to blame for having created them. Even the most cooperative and "psychologically minded" patients may not be willing to reveal critical data until they have developed some feeling of trust and respect for the physician.

Finally, the physician should be aware that, by virtue of personality traits or cultural influences, some people are just not good communicators. Not everyone in our society adheres to the belief that one's mental health is enhanced by sharing personal experiences with others. Some patients may avoid self-disclosure simply because they are unaccustomed to talking about themselves, or because they cannot perceive how self-disclosure may be relevant to their illness or their treatment.

Often, even a skilled clinician is unaware that the patient is withholding information. Clinicians who do long-term psychotherapy (therapy that continues for months or years) are very familiar with situations in which patients suddenly reveal some previously unsuspected but vital information about themselves, many weeks, months, or years after treatment has been initiated. Some of my patients have failed to report financial problems, previous illnesses, drug abuse, criminal behavior, extramarital affairs, and paraphiliac tendencies until months of treatment have elapsed. Other patients have covered up hallucinatory experiences and delusional ideas for months or longer. I once treated a patient for over five years without knowing she was delusional. When nearing termination of psychotherapy, this highly intelligent and successful person told me that she believed I had been surreptitiously hypnotizing her from the first day of treatment. Over the years, she had come to believe that I was doing it for benevolent reasons, and she believed that she had been greatly helped by her treatment. At the point of termination, she felt well enough and safe enough with me to chide me for not having been more direct about using hypnosis.

WHY DO PATIENTS SOMETIMES PROVIDE INACCURATE INFORMATION?

In most aspects of medical practice, the physician anticipates that patients will be truthful. It is assumed that some patients will deny or exaggerate symptomatology, but that intentional distortion of data will rarely occur. This assumption should not be made with psychiatric patients. Because of the frightening nature of mental illness and its possible social consequences, some psychiatric patients not only withhold information but deliberately present an inaccurate picture of their history and experiences to the evaluator. Psychiatric patients are also more likely than other patients to deliberately exaggerate symptomatology in an effort to elicit attention or nurturant responses from the physician. Patients who are evaluated for agencies (such as insurers or employers) may believe (at times correctly) that truthfulness is not in their best interest. Although psychiatrists cannot afford to be too cynical about the accuracy of patient-generated information, they should also avoid naiveté. Some of the most serious errors in diagnosis and treatment occur when the psychiatrist uncritically accepts the truthfulness of the patient's communication.

Patients may resort to dishonesty if they are asked directly about something they do not wish to reveal. A young man may be embarrassed by his lack of sexual experience and lie about it when asked. A young woman may be too ashamed to discuss her sexual activities (particularly if the evaluator is a male physician); even if her sexual activities are a source of great anguish to her, she may deceptively insist that she has no problems. A similar type of dishonesty is common in those who have substance-abuse or eating disorders, and *who tend to exaggerate or minimize* the extent of their problems. These patients may try to deceive themselves as well as others by ignoring or trivializing the extent of their loss of control.

When patients have difficulty behaving in a socially acceptable manner because of severe emotional or cognitive disturbances, they may wish to hide their difficulties from the evaluator. Often they cannot do this very well and, instead, resort to dishonest communication. They may try to explain previous aberrant behavior on the basis of confabulated facts that make that behavior appear more rational. A patient who withdraws from social contacts because of great interpersonal anxiety or delusional fears of harm may explain such isolation as an effort to obtain rest and privacy. Or a patient who turns up the volume on the stereo to drown out auditory hallucinations may insist that she or he merely wishes to enjoy some good music.

Patients who experience memory loss may be especially concerned about hiding this fact from others. Often, they try to create a new reality or a fictitious set of remembrances to help account for the memory lapse. Such fictitious memories or confabulations may be so bizarre as to make the evaluator immediately aware that these patients have some type of disorder. Although it is never entirely clear whether patients believe their confabulations, such communications can be viewed as a form of self-protective dishonesty.

When patients present with symptoms that are ordinarily associated with organic dysfunction but that turn out to have no organic basis, or when they present with symptoms that are ordinarily associated with psychiatric disorders but that appear to be factitious or exaggerated, they are likely to be categorized as having some type of psychiatric disorder, usually a factitious or somatoform disorder. Some patients who are diagnosed as having factitious disorders may deliberately fabricate symptoms with the only apparent goal being assuming the role of patient. Other patients, diagnosed as having personality disorders or somatoform disorders, appear to create new symptoms or to exaggerate older ones without an awareness that they are doing so. Their escalation of symptomatology is not intentional, nor do they perceive it as something they can control.

It is usually difficult to understand why patients would voluntarily or involuntarily seek to create or exaggerate symptoms when such behavior provides them no apparent gratification. A common assumption is that these symptoms develop in order to help the patient gain the attention and nurturance of loved ones or medical personnel. There is a difference between this group of patients and those who deliberately simulate symptoms in order to achieve some obvious goal, such as receiving disability rewards or avoiding military service. The latter group are ordinarily viewed not as sick but as malingerers.

Another group of patients who tend to exaggerate symptoms are those who suffer from serious depression. In addition to having many somatic complaints, depressed patients may also complain of psychiatric symptomatology, such as memory loss or inability to concentrate, which suggests the presence of organic brain disease. When tested carefully, these patients turn out to have no actual impairment of their cognitive capacities. For this reason, their symptom presentation is sometimes described as *pseudodementia*. It is unclear why depressed patients act this way. One explanation is that depression is associated with an enormous fear of loss of capacity, and that depressed patients eventually come to believe that their fears have been realized. It may also be true that depressed patients exaggerate or simulate symptomatology in order to communicate the severity of their despair to the physician, actually an extreme form of attention or nurturance seeking.

Patients with personality disorders (especially antisocial and histrionic personalities), in addition to exaggerating or creating symptoms, may provide false information in order to gain some social or interpersonal advantage. Particularly when institutionalized, these patients may have great difficulty in relating honestly to authority figures. Sometimes, such patients feel that they can keep authority figures (including physicians) "off their backs" by telling them only what they want to hear. At other times, these patients may feel that, by providing false information, they are gaining power over their physician. Adolescents who feel alienated from the adult world may be similarly deceptive. In general, all patients who are reluctantly or involuntarily evaluated tend to provide false information, particularly when they feel oppressed by or distrustful of those who hold power over them.

Finally, there are situations in which patients may find quite tangible advantages in being dishonest. The patient who is seeking disability payments or an excuse from an obligation such as military service may exaggerate symptomatology. On the other hand, the patient who is seeking to retain or obtain a privilege, such as professional licensure or a job, will minimize symptomatology. Patients involved in custody disputes may deliberately exaggerate both their own virtues and the weaknesses of their spouses. Patients who want to resist civil commitment will perceive themselves as benefiting by denying symptoms that suggest suicidal or homicidal feelings and by confabulating apparently rational explanations of past deviant behavior. Patients who are litigants will be tempted to distort information in order to present themselves in a manner that favors their legal needs. It is not uncommon in forensic work for plaintiffs in personal injury cases or defendants in criminal cases to present themselves as very disturbed when examined by psychiatrists whom their attorneys have employed. On the other hand, they may reveal very little to the psychiatrist employed by the other party, who is perceived as a potential adversary. In my own experience, I have found patients to be especially suspicious and withholding when they are involved in personal injury suits and I am evaluating them for the defense.

Most of the above examples of dishonest communication are intentional and occur in situations where patients are likely to be aware of exaggeration of distortion. (The exception is patients with somatoform disorders and possibly depressed patients who show pseudodementia.) Clinicians must also be aware of other situations in which patients distort information without being aware that they are doing so. Remote memories are especially prone to distortion. Many people tend to recall the past in ways that explain, rationalize, or justify the present. As a reaction to grief, a deceased loved one may be overidealized. Parents may be falsely idealized or falsely devalued. The significance of stresses may be minimized or exaggerated. Family myths of specialness are also likely to be perpetuated. Where family members are available, it is easier to check on the accuracy of the patient's past history. Otherwise, the clinician must simply learn to keep an open mind about the accuracy of the patient's reporting of historical events; where the reporting seems to explain or justify the patient's situation too facilely, the clinician should be especially skeptical.

WHAT FACTORS MAXIMIZE THE EXTENT AND ACCURACY OF THE PATIENT'S COMMUNICATIONS?

One of the main factors that influences the willingness of patients to communicate fully and accurately is their desire to be relieved of painful symptoms. The extent and quality of this desire is in turn determined by the degree of distress they are experiencing. One of the most complex aspects of mental illness is that the level of discomfort it produces is not consistent over time. Often, patients can control or modify the severity of their mental anguish by drastically altering their patterns of behaving or thinking. An obvious example of this phenomenon is found in the agoraphobic patient, who may be quite comfortable as long as he or she leads a seclusive life. Indeed, so long as this isolation is tolerable, such a patient may not wish to seek help. A less obvious example is the psychotic patient who deals with the terror of being unable to remember or to think clearly by developing and clinging to a belief system that some other person is deliberately causing this impairment. Here, the patient "defends" against pain caused by a loss of vital cognitive functions by drastically altering the accuracy of his or her thinking. Such patients may be viewed as disturbed by observers, but as long as they can sustain their "defenses," these patients may not appreciate a need for help and may approach the psychiatric evaluation with little motivation to cooperate.

The beginning psychiatrist is often tempted to attack the reliance of some patients on pain-diminishing avoidance or distortion in the hope of increasing their motivation. This approach is generally ill advised. The mandate of physicians is to alleviate pain and suffering. If they try to do anything to increase pain and suffering in order to motivate the patient, there is a risk that the patient will respond by avoiding a new source of pain (i.e., the physician) and by becoming even less willing to cooperate. There is also the serious ethical question of whether physicians should temporarily try to induce more psychic pain in a patient in the hope that it will serve the ultimate good of curing the patient. In certain forms of long-term psychotherapy with patients who have personality disorders or in the behavioral therapy of phobic disorders, there may well be a place for techniques of confrontation or frustration that temporarily increase the anxiety of patients. But these techniques are most appropriately used with patients who know what to expect and who have contracted to participate in a form of therapy that is likely to increase anxiety.

Fortunately, there are factors other than the patient's motivation to be freed from suffering that will enhance the patient's communication and that the physician has a greater capacity to influence. One obvious determinant of this kind is the patient's belief that the physician can be helpful. Patients are more likely to view interactions with the physician as potentially helpful when they have the capacity to conceptualize their troubling behavior or troubling thoughts and feelings as a form of mental illness. Many psychiatric patients do not view themselves as having mental disorders. To the extent that they believe that their symptoms are an appropriate response to social oppression or that these symptoms represent criminal or sinful tendencies, they may be less willing to see them as manifestations of illness. Here, the physician has the opportunity to explain to patients how deviant behavior and perceptions can be conceptualized as illness, and how they may be helped through medical intervention. Even if patients accept their distress as a form of illness, however, they may still be unconvinced that medical science, and particularly psychiatric medicine, can help them. Here, the clinician is faced with the task of communicating to patients an optimistic but realistic picture of the extent to which psychiatric disorders can be alleviated or cured.

Even if patients view their symptoms as manifestations of an illness and believe that medical science can help them, they may still not appreciate the need to maximize the amount of information presented to the physician. Many patients are accustomed to viewing themselves as passive participants in the process of evaluation. They may present their symptoms to the doctor, answer a few questions, and then wait for the doctor to perform examinations and tests that will tell the doctor what is wrong with them. They are then willing to do whatever the doctor tells them to do in order to get better. In effect, this is the "standard" model of participation in medical care. Unfortunately, it is unlikely to be effective in psychiatry—although at the outset, the patient cannot be expected to know this. Most patients have to be educated about the complexity of psychiatric disorders and about how their accurate diagnosis and effective treatment depend on maximizing communication. Much of this educative process can be accomplished during the course of evaluation. The physician can inform the patient repeatedly that many factors contribute to the development, the course, and the treatment of a psychiatric illness and that the process of information collection must cover a much broader range of issues than the patient has been accustomed to dealing with in previous doctor–patient interactions.

If patients are to reveal information that they feel may reflect adversely on them, they must have some assurance that their revelations will not be used to harm them. Patients can perceive themselves as harmed if private information is shared with others, including family, friends, or social agencies. Such sharing may indeed cause them embarrassment, may threaten their relationships, or may lead to a curtailment of privileges. In most evaluative situations, the physician can honestly reassure the patient of sufficient confidentiality to allow the patient to communicate freely without fear of harm. The patient, of course, must be convinced that the physician is telling the truth. Although some sophisticated patients have a good idea of the extent of the confidentiality that psychiatrists provide, most patients do not. It is always useful for the psychiatrist to inform the patient of the limits of confidentiality as early in the interview as possible. Where the psychiatrist is agency-employed and information is likely to be shared with others, the patient is best informed of this fact before the interview begins. Ordinarily, such honesty on the part of the physician will enhance rather than diminish communication, particularly where the patient is aware of the physician's double-agent role and appreciates his or her honesty.

Perhaps the most important factor in promoting the communication, one that the physician can certainly influence, is the patient's level of comfort during the interview. Patients are the most likely to communicate when they feel the least anxiety. One way of conceptualizing this helpful factor is in terms of the kind of interview environment the psychiatrist creates for the patient. Assuming that they do not have personality traits that somehow diminish communication with a particular patient, experienced evaluators should be able to create an interview climate in which patients feel so comfortable that they are willing and even eager to communicate. Such an environment enhances patients' immediate sense of well-being and prepares the way for future positive interaction; in particular, these qualities allow the environment to be characterized as therapeutic or facilitative. Much of psychiatric training is directed toward maximizing the physician's capacity to create a therapeutic or facilitative environment.

HOW CAN THE PHYSICIAN CREATE A THERAPEUTIC OR FACILITATIVE ENVIRONMENT DURING THE PROCESS OF EVALUATION?

The answer to this question is what much of this book is about; in subsequent chapters, this subject will be discussed in relation to a variety of specific issues. Here, only the general attitudinal and technical aspects of facilitating communication are considered.

The Evaluation Setting

Ideally, patients should be evaluated in a setting that maximizes their comfort. There should be more than one chair available to the patient, preferably at varying distances from the physician, which give patients some choice in how physically close they may wish to be to the evaluator. Care must be taken that the evaluator's chair is no higher than the patient's, so that the patient does not feel overwhelmed by the authority of the physician. The lighting should be subdued; the surroundings might well include books, works of art, or plants; and all in all, the setting should be as pleasant as possible. Soundproofing, of course, is desirable, and background noise should be minimal.

The beginning student or resident may view all of the above suggestions as absurd or unrealistic. Patients may have to be evaluated in a hospital room or ward where the setting is stark and uncomfortable, and where privacy is at best partial. Even the outpatient resident may be assigned an office so cramped that he or she can barely avoid touching the patient if either makes an unexpected move. (For several years after I began work at my current position, I wondered why the male residents I supervised reported so little sexual material in their treatment of female patients. It was not until I took a careful look at their offices that I realized that it would be very difficult for a patient to discuss sex with a therapist of the opposite sex when their knees are almost touching.) There is not much the resident can do about this situation except to be aware that communication will be compromised if conditions are not optimal. When examining hospitalized patients who are ambulatory, the resident or the medical student should also make realistic efforts to seek a comfortable and private office.

The Physician's Appearance

It is helpful for physicians to dress and groom in such a manner that they look something like the patient's image of how a physician *should* look. If patients are to view their disturbances as a manifestation of illness and are to have confidence that their suffering can be alleviated by medical science, it helps for them to have a firm idea that the evaluator is indeed a doctor—or soon to become one. Patients, of course, differ in their images of the doctor. Elderly patients may be comforted by the white coat of the physician. Most middle-aged patients expect their doctors to be conservatively dressed (ties for men, dresses or skirts and blouses for women), and younger patients may be comfortable with a physician who is dressed more casually. The evaluator obviously cannot fit each generational or socioeconomic class image. However, in dealing with patients of different ages and socioeconomic class (such as one finds on a general hospital psychiatric ward), the physician will offend the fewest people by dressing conservatively. Good grooming is, of course, mandatory. All generations will perceive the sloppily dressed, uncombed or unclean physician as fatigued, deviant, or uninterested in the patient's problem.

Maximizing the Patient's Dignity

There are inherent inequalities in power between doctor and patient. The doctor's knowledge of disease and healing gives him or her the power to satisfy what the patient may perceive to be desperate needs. Frequently, patients feel so needy and helpless that they are willing to sacrifice the autonomy they might normally seek in other personal relationships. In situations where patients must sacrifice autonomy (or the capacity to choose their own course of action), they are also at the risk of losing dignity. They are especially vulnerable to invasions of privacy, such as being asked personal questions or submitting to physical procedures that in any other setting would be considered indignities. At the same time, if they are to feel enough comfort and trust to communicate accurately, it is necessary that patients sustain a proper level of dignity.

One way of maximizing this sense of dignity is to allow the patient as much self-determination or autonomy as possible in the interview setting. Although the physician will want some power to influence the patient, that power should never be greater than that which is justified by the doctor's superior knowledge and skills. Even in making decisions related to diagnosis and treatment, it is best for the physician to view the patient as an individual of full worth. That is to say, as long as they are competent, patients have full power to control their actions in the evaluative process. In practice, that means that a competent patient's refusal to respond to a question or even a refusal to participate in the evaluation should be honored. The physician may want to explain the consequences of noncooperation to the reluctant patient but should never force the patient to cooperate. Respect for the patient's autonomy is also implied in the physician's willingness to answer questions that the patient may ask (and that are answerable). In general, physicians should be willing to share any knowledge of the patient's condition with the patient, unless they have good reason to believe that such sharing will influence the patient adversely.

A related issue is the willingness of physicians to share with the patient information about themselves. Patients may ask about the physician's background, experience, or personal value system. Some of these questions may be offensive to the evaluator, or they may represent patients' efforts to divert attention from themselves. Here, the evaluator may be reluctant to respond. In settings where psychoanalytic theories of treatment are emphasized, clinicians may be advised to reveal as little of themselves as possible in order to remain a "blank screen" and to expedite "transference." My own views are that, most of the time, little harm is done and information flow is facilitated when the physician answers reasonable questions. The judgment about which questions are offensive, distracting, or, if answered, likely to compromise the process of treatment is, of course, a difficult one. When the evaluator feels that a question should not be answered, efforts can be made to preserve the patient's dignity with a response such as one of the following:

> I may be wrong, but it seems that there is a lot of anger implied in your question. Before I try to respond, it might be helpful for us to consider whether I am right. If I am, can we talk about your anger?
>
> The question you are asking me is quite personal, and I don't think answering it would be helpful to you. I hope you don't mind my not responding to it until I know you better.
>
> I have a feeling that you are asking me questions to avoid answering mine. I don't mind answering your questions, but please tell me if my questions are making you uncomfortable.
>
> I can speculate about the reasons why you are asking this question, but if I am to understand you, it would help me to know what your reasons are.
>
> I'll be glad to answer your questions, but I wonder if you would first tell me what you anticipate my answer will be.

The student should be reminded that the patient does not always appreciate the reasons why evaluators may not want to reveal information about themselves. There is always a risk that the patient will experience the evaluator's refusal as rudeness, and this perception will impair communication. This risk is minimized if the evaluator provides cogent reasons for not responding.

Another way in which the therapist maximizes the patient's autonomy and dignity is by ascertaining whether the patient knows of any risks that may result from frank communication. Patients are certainly at risk of being harmed when they are evaluated by agency-employed psychiatrists. They are also at some risk when they seek treatment in situations where complete confidentiality cannot be fully guaranteed. When patients pay for treatment through insurers, the fact of their seeing a psychiatrist is known by many people. If they seek future licensing as professionals, they may have to reveal the fact of their previous psychiatric treatment to a certification board. Informing patients of these risks may certainly cause some to reveal less than they otherwise might; on the other hand, it may also facilitate communication. In my experience, most patients quickly develop trust in a doctor who is willing to be truthful. The doctor's honesty is always a powerful statement of acknowledgment of the patient's worth.

Still another minor but important way in which the evaluator can maximize patients' dignity is by addressing them by their proper title or last name. There is a distressing tendency on the part of beginners in the mental health field to assume that rapport and intimacy are generated when patients are called by their first names. Sometimes, beginners even use this form of address in communicating with an individual who is much older than they are. There may be times when it is appropriate for doctors and patients to call one another by their first names, but the evaluation interview is certainly not one of them. The patient has already lost some dignity in assuming a help-seeking role. Being immediately referred to by one's first name is usually infantilizing and often degrading.

Emphasizing the Need for Communication

One way in which the physician helps the patient to understand the need for optimal communication is simply to tell the patient about it. Statements such as the following may be provided early in the interview: "I have to try to understand your problems before I can recommend treatment. To do that, I will spend more time asking you questions and listening and talking to you than most other doctors do. It is important that you tell me everything about your symptoms that you can. It is also important that you try to answer my questions as accurately as you can.

If it seems that some of my questions are too personal or unrelated to your problem, tell me, and I'll try to explain why I'm asking them."

Another way in which the evaluator indicates the need for information is by the comprehensiveness of the questions. When patients report symptoms such as headache, for example, the evaluator may ask them to describe it in great detail, offering various adjectives such as *throbbing*, *sharp*, or *dull* to assist them in providing accurate descriptions. The evaluator will also want to know the location of a headache, what time of day it occurs, how long it lasts, whether other symptoms are associated with it, how often it occurs, when it first began, what alleviates it, how it influences other aspects of the patient's behavior, and if any events, thoughts, or bodily feelings precede or follow it. This kind of thorough delineating of the nature of the patient's symptomatology gives the patient some idea of the depth of information the evaluator is going to seek. As the physician continues to demonstrate an unrelenting concern with detail, the patient will usually try to help by presenting comprehensive information in a more spontaneous manner.

Diminishing the Patient's Anxiety

Any aspect of the interview environment that makes the patient feel understood and valued tends to relieve the patient's anxiety. The manner in which the evaluator tries to communicate understanding and respect for the patient will be discussed in the next section. Other techniques for diminishing the patient's anxiety are considered here.

Whatever problems the patient may have with being anxious in other interpersonal settings may well be exacerbated in the psychiatric interview. Patients may fear the immediate consequences of demonstrating the depth of their disability to another person, of being told that their condition is not treatable, or of being rejected by the evaluator. They may also fear the subsequent consequences of losing freedom or other privileges as a result of the evaluation. The evaluator can minimize much of the patient's fear of rejection by being attentive and thorough in the process of history taking. It is especially important to avoid judgmental responses. When patients expect to be blamed for behavior, thoughts, or feelings, they are pleasantly relieved when they are not.

Patients' fears of being told they are incurable or of having something done to them coercively can often be modified by the evaluator's making positive statements such as "It did get better before," "It sounds as if that medicine really does help you," or "You seem to have handled your serious stresses very well." A somewhat more subtle way of accomplishing the same goal is to ask questions that imply that the patient will have a symptom-free future, such as "What are some of the things you want to do that you can't do now?" and "What are your plans for the future?" A still more subtle way of communicating optimism is to imply that patients have some control over their symptoms by asking questions such as "How would you like to improve your relationship with your spouse?" or "Can you think of anything you can do to help you cope with these stresses?"

(The student must be warned about some important exceptions. Some severely depressed or psychotic patients will already have communicated a sense of hopelessness or helplessness; they are then likely to perceive such future-oriented or autonomy-inducing questions as insensitive.)

Perhaps the most important techniques available to the physician are those that help patients maintain a sense that, during the interview, they are in control of their behavior, thoughts, and feelings. It is one thing for patients to talk about their symptoms. However embarrassing this may be, in their interaction with the evaluator patients who are describing their problems are still exercising some self-control. It is something entirely different for patients to demonstrate symptoms by revealing their inability to conduct themselves appropriately, to organize their thinking, or to remember. Some patients, particularly those with personality disorders, may intend to demonstrate rather than talk about their symptoms. The majority of patients who display symptomatology during the interview, however, do not wish to do so; moreover, they are often sufficiently aware of what they are doing to be humiliated by the fact that this is happening. The physician usually seeks to minimize the patient's tendency to demonstrate symptoms. This approach, in turn, is likely to maximize the patient's ability to talk about his or her symptoms.

Beginners often question why they should try to keep the demonstration of symptoms to a minimum during an interview. They presume that observing the patient's symptomatic behavior will provide a more objective picture of the presenting problem than hearing the patient talk about it. In medical school, they learned a great deal about illness by observing their teachers ask, allow, or encourage patients to demonstrate their pathology. Moreover, they may have seen their psychiatric teachers interview patients and elicit symptomatic responses that aided in the diagnostic process. The student is also aware that parts of the mental status examination can be viewed as tests that are designed to demonstrate the patient's incapacities. It must indeed be acknowledged that the diagnostic process is often enhanced when patients display their symptoms. Yet, I believe that the benefit of enhancing patient's sense of control by diminishing the degree to which they present symptoms usually outweighs the diagnostic advantages when symptoms are expressed. One reason for this belief is that, early in the interview, no matter what the evaluator does, sicker patients usually manifest a certain amount of symptomatology. Once such pathology is seen, it does not have to be repeatedly observed in order for the physician to make a diagnosis. Less disturbed patients can usually describe their symptoms accurately, and there is little to be gained by having those symptoms demonstrated.

(It is important to note that it is a little easier for patients to reveal incapacities in the course of a formal mental status examination. This is a time-limited procedure in which patients know they are being tested. For most people, failure on a test is not nearly as humiliating as failure to behave rationally or to adhere to accepted roles of social conduct. Even in test situations, however, patients should not be allowed to demonstrate too much of the incapacities that might embarrass them.)

Another compelling reason for trying to strengthen the patient's sense of control is to maximize the physician's safety. The clinician is especially concerned that the patient talk about rather than demonstrate anger. With some patients, the demonstration of anger can quickly be followed by violence.

Perhaps the main exception to the technical stance I am advocating occurs when the evaluator feels that the patient is successfully covering up a powerful emotion that needs therapeutic discussion, but that will not be approached unless the patient is allowed to identify it during the interview. Patients may not discuss feelings of sadness or anger unless they experience and disclose them. Some examples of comments that elicit this kind of symptomatology are "You've been through so much, you must be sad," "You seem to be very sad," or "You look as if you're trying to prevent yourself from showing me how angry you feel." These statements are designed to help the patient to experience and discuss feelings, and not necessarily to express them.

The interviewer can influence the extent to which the patient exposes symptomatology during the interview by controlling both the content and the form of questions. Severely incapacitated patients have trouble discussing certain topics; they become so anxious that they get confused. This may be especially true in the early part of the interview, before the patient feels any degree of trust in the physician. As a rule, any subject that reflects unfavorably on patients or that may expose their pathology before they are ready to address it will elicit anxious responses. When the interviewer senses that his or her questions are disturbing the patient and causing the patient to demonstrate too much pathology, the easiest course is to change the subject. Usually, switching to topics that are relatively neutral, such as past history or family history, will allow patients to regain control and present themselves more rationally. This technique is especially useful with psychotic patients, as the following incident illustrates.

Several years ago, while serving as an examiner for the American

Board of Psychiatry and Neurology, I observed a candidate begin an interview with a young male patient by inquiring about his symptoms. The patient quickly went off on a tangent and angrily began a disjointed account of how he had been mistreated throughout his life. He soon turned his anger against the candidate. When the candidate persisted in asking about the patient's symptoms, the patient became even angrier and refused to respond to the examiner's questions. Finally, the patient turned to me and insisted that he had to go to the bathroom. The other examiner and I were eager to break up this painful situation and give both the patient and the candidate a chance to start over. We agreed that I would escort the patient to a nearby bathroom and then bring him back. As the patient and I began walking to the bathroom, I asked him where he was from. He replied coherently, and we continued to have an informative and rational two-minute conversation about his hometown. When he returned to the examination room, the candidate again began asking the patient about symptoms. The patient again became mute. The candidate failed the examination.

During an interview with an impaired patient, there may be many instances in which the clinician is well advised to back off from sensitive material. The patient may develop anxious responses even when talking about events that appear innocuous to the examiner. When formally testing cognitive functions during the course of the mental status examination, the physician may also have to be careful not to overstress the patient. The patient needs to feel a sense of success during the interview and should never be allowed to wallow in failures. If the patient fails to repeat five numbers backward, it is usually harmful to ask him to repeat five numbers backward again. Some patients become very disturbed when they are unable to provide correct responses to the examiner's questions. This possibility is diminished when the examiner begins testing cognitive functions by asking questions that the patient is likely to answer correctly.

Patients who are having difficulty organizing their thoughts also respond most coherently to clear and unambiguous questions presented in a logical fashion. It is relatively easy (but usually unwarranted) for the clinician to elicit symptomatology by asking questions that are vague or by shifting the topic too rapidly. Even certain types of questions that are common in other aspects of medical evaluation may be difficult for mentally incapacitated patients. There are times when questions such as "What brings you here?" or "How can I help you?" or "How are you doing?" will overwhelm the capacities of psychiatric patients.

Interview questions can be divided into the categories of open-ended or closed-ended. Open-ended questions require a creative and sometimes complex response. They include questions such as "How do you feel?" and "What do you plan to do next?" and "How do you explain what is happening to you?" Closed-ended questions can be answered with a simple phrase. The patient either knows or does not know the answer; creativity is not involved. Some examples of closed-ended questions are "How old are you?" and "Where do you live?" and "Are you married?" With highly incapacitated patients, it is often useful to limit the number of open-ended questions asked and to ask more closed-ended questions. As the latter are more easily answered, they are used to increase the patient's sense of making a successful presentation of himself or herself and to diminish anxiety.

In concluding this section, it is worth reemphasizing that, during the interview, skilled clinicians use more energy trying to make the patient look healthy than they do in trying to elicit pathology. There is great satisfaction for all parties involved when patients are able to present a comprehensive picture of their difficulties without being subjected to feelings of humiliation and dyscontrol.

Helping the Patient Feel Understood

Patients are most likely to communicate freely when they feel that the doctor understands their thoughts and feelings or is at least trying very hard to understand them. Being understood by a sympathetic listener is often anxiety-relieving in itself. It is also a powerful sign that the doctor will be able to help the patient. This is particularly true when the doctor communicates understanding in a compassionate way by showing feelings of concern for the patient's suffering and a desire to be helpful. If the doctor continues to come across as an understanding and caring person, or at least as one who is trying to be understanding and caring, the patient's level of trust in the doctor will increase. As patients' trust, safety, and optimism with regard to the evaluative situation increase, they will be more willing to share information about themselves. (The above observations are true for most patients most of the time. However, it is worth remembering that, at times, some patients are fearful of being understood. And there are always the few who have dishonest motives in seeking evaluation and who do not wish to be understood. In short, there are at least a few situations in which the physician will not wish to let patients know the extent to which they may be understood.)

There are many factors involved in determining whether patients are understood, including their ability to communicate their thoughts and feelings accurately. The most important factors, however, are the physician's capacity to resonate with the patient's experience or, in brief, to be empathic. *Empathy* refers to the process of putting oneself in the psychological frame of reference of another, so that the other person's experiences, thinking, and feeling are understood. Physicians' level of empathy is directly related to the extent to which they can ask themselves and imagine, "What is it like being this person?" Empathy in itself is a useful tool in understanding the patient's problem and in making a diagnosis. If it is to be used to catalyze the communication process, however, it must be expressed to the patient. Empathic skills involve more than just understanding the patient; they also include the capacity to know how and when to communicate that understanding.

It is likely that the most important skills one learns in medical and psychiatric training are the ability to be empathic and to communicate empathy. Some clinicians may be born with greater capacities to empathize than others. Obviously, the greater the breadth of one's own experience, the greater is one's capacity to identify with the experience of others. For this reason, to have been a patient oneself or at least to have role-played the role of patient is helpful. Many kinds of experiences can help the clinician develop empathic skills, for example, learning experiences outside psychiatric training involving interaction with other people or observation of other people by reading or by viewing movies or plays. The chief means by which empathic skills are developed in medicine, however, is for the clinician to seek constantly the sense of what the patient is experiencing, and then to check the accuracy of that conjecture by observing the patient's subsequent communications and behavior. As these interactions are repeated thousands of times, as mistakes are corrected by teachers, and particularly as the clinician develops more certainty about conjectures by following selected patients for long periods of time, the capacity for empathy gradually improves. If this does not happen, the clinician is well advised to leave the profession of psychiatry.

When students ask how they can become more empathic, the most realistic advice is that they should interview as many patients as possible under the supervision of the best teachers available, to read as much as possible (poetry, fiction, and especially biography), to know themselves, and to lead a full life. Above all, the student should never stop asking, "What is it like to be this patient?"

When it comes to the skill of communicating empathy, more specific advice can be given. The question of *when* empathy should be communicated is best resolved by the admonition, "Whenever the clinician feels that he or she actually does understand the patient's experience and believes that the patient will be comforted by knowing that such understanding is present." The question of *how* empathy is communicated is more complex. There are several skills involved here, all of which can be studied and developed during the course of psychiatric training.

Perhaps the most effective way of showing empathy or compassionate understanding is by nonverbal means. Such variables as facial expression, the intensity of posture, hand movements, and even head nodding communicate a great deal about the physician's level of understanding and concern. Often, beginning clinicians are unaware of how their facial expressions or body language changes when they are empathic, but anyone observing the interview usually knows when they are "on target." With repeated self-observation and feedback from others, experienced clinicians become ever more aware of the nonverbal cues they emit and learn to use them to communicate empathy. They can be very empathic while saying very little. For patients who have become distrustful of the spoken word, body language that communicates compassionate understanding is often more reassuring than any verbal statements that the physician can make.

The physician's questions can communicate empathy. One important way in which the physician indicates willingness to understand is by the thoroughness of questioning, particularly with regard to the patient's feelings and degree of suffering. Questions can be asked such as "How did you feel when he ignored you?" or "How do you usually deal with people who are rude to you?" There is a clear implication that the evaluator already has some idea of what the answer will be and is concerned about the severity of the patient's distress or disability. Sometimes, such questions get directly to the essence of the patient's feeling. The evaluator who asks, "Did you feel some anger then?" or "Were you embarrassed?" is already indicating some awareness of the patient's feeling state. By asking questions in a manner that communicates understanding and concern, the clinician not only gains more data but concurrently expedites the process by which data are collected.

Sometimes, the clinician can demonstrate understanding and at the same time help patients develop a clearer picture of their experience. This can be done by providing an interpretation of the patient's behavior or feeling. Statements such as "Perhaps you are angry" or "I wonder if you are feeling sad" communicate the clinician's awareness of emotional states that the patient may have trouble identifying. The clinician who is correct helps patients understand themselves while communicating his or her own understanding.

Finally, the evaluator may wish to use direct expressions of compassion and understanding by making statements such as "You must have felt really awful," "You must really suffer when that happens," or "I can understand how bad you feel." Such direct expressions of the physician's understanding and concern can have a powerful impact. The physician is cautioned, however, to be aware of certain pitfalls in the use of such statements. First, if the physician is incorrect in gauging the patient's experiences and communicates this false perception, the patient may lose confidence in him or her. Second, words of comfort and understanding are often distrusted by the patient. By the time psychiatric patients have reached the physician, they are likely to have heard many such remarks from friends and family members and to have found them kind, but not helpful. Experienced clinicians rely more on nonverbal behavior, questioning, and interpretation than on direct expression of empathy. The direct expression of empathy is best used sparingly, primarily in situations where there is a high probability that the clinician's perceptions are at once accurate and likely to be perceived as sincerely felt.

Using Operant Conditioning in the Evaluative Process

The psychiatric interview is an interaction between two parties in which each has the opportunity to shape the behavior of the other. Patients can affect the nature of the interviewer's responses by withholding or distorting information or by failing to adhere to the ordinary rules of conversation. (This happens when the patient becomes mute, violent, amorous, or belligerent or otherwise behaves inappropriately.) Ultimately, however, because the physician is less needy and more powerful in the doctor–patient relationship, he or she should be able to control how the interaction is defined. The physician generally uses principles of behavior modification (whether these responses are thought of as behavior modification or not) to create a climate in which patients receive a clear understanding of what is expected of them and also experience reinforcement if they maximize communication.

During the interview, the interviewer can usually prevent inappropriate behavior by reminding the patient that their interactions will be primarily verbal. Patients who suggest some type of physical contact, whether it be amorous or belligerent, should be reminded that such behavior is not acceptable. This reminder tells patients that, if any physical actions take place, they risk the probably aversive response of the interview's being ended.

The physician can also limit the presentation of repetitive or irrelevant material by failing to show interest in it and by asking questions that direct the patient to other issues. If patients repeatedly emphasize their helplessness and misery, for example, and seem unable to talk about anything else, the clinician may try to limit such communication by saying, "I think you have done a good job of acquainting me with the extent of your suffering, and I now know how bad things are. If I'm going to help you, however, I need to learn about other things. Perhaps you can tell me how your wife responds to you when you are so unhappy." In this kind of maneuver, the patient is not reinforced for talking about suffering and is instead cued to the possibility that talking about other issues may lead to subsequent reinforcement. At the same time, the clinician is using the behavioral process of extinction to decrease the frequency of unwanted responses by failing to reinforce them.

The physician can increase the likelihood that the patient will talk about more relevant issues by providing positive reinforcement when this happens, by communicating a sense of compassion or concern and by indicating through facial expression and questioning a high level of interest in certain communications. Sometimes, the clinician may reinforce the patient by making such supportive statements as "That's a very clear description" or "You're doing a very good job of helping me understand a very complex situation." The clinician is generally highly reinforcing and nonjudgmental (nonpunishing) when the patient brings up unpleasant feelings. Here, the patient may be ashamed and embarrassed and may fear some type of rejecting comment from the physician. If the interviewer responds with a compassionate response, such as "It must be very difficult for you to talk about this, but I'm glad you can tell me about these feelings," the patient will feel reinforced and will be more willing to discuss painful feelings. In general, successful psychiatrists tend to be liberal in reinforcing patients who are cooperating in the evaluative process. Such clinicians also try to diminish noncooperative behavior or irrelevant communication by simply not reinforcing it. They do not resort to aversive responsives unless the patient is threatening to disrupt the interview.

IN SUMMARY, WHAT ARE THE MAIN ISSUES THAT CLINICIANS SHOULD CONSIDER AS THEY TRY TO MAXIMIZE PATIENT COMMUNICATION?

1. Although there is a natural tendency on the part of all of us to want to believe that people are accurate reporters of internal and external events, psychiatrists must learn that much of the information they receive is inaccurate. An awareness of the possibility of inaccuracy discourages psychiatrists from assuming a premature understanding of the patient's problem. It also encourages them to ask more questions and to dig deeply into issues even if this process involves some repetitiveness.

2. It is rarely useful (or ethically justifiable) to put stress on patients in order to get them to reveal pathology. Rather, physicians need to spend more time explaining to patients the need to provide information, and explaining why so many detailed questions are necessary.

3. Patients should be provided with as much confidentiality as is possible within the social context of the evaluation and should be informed of the limits of confidentiality.

4. Everything about the environment in which the assessment takes place and everything about the evaluative process should be structured so as to enhance the patient's sense of dignity and self-esteem. For highly disturbed patients, techniques may be required that diminish the

degree of pathology they demonstrate and that enhance their sense of success in the interview.

5. Physicians should constantly strive to put themselves in their patients' shoes. This is a never-ending exercise. When physicians feel that they understand the patient, it is generally helpful to communicate this understanding to the patient.

6. Communication is generally facilitated by providing clear instructions to the patient about what type of information is being sought and then reinforcing the patient when such information is provided. Physicians who provide a high level of positive reinforcement to their patients are generally good history takers.

FOR FURTHER READING

Bird, B. *Talking with patients*. Lippincott, Philadelphia, 1973.

Enelow, A. J., and Swisher, S. N. *Interviewing and patient care*. Oxford University Press, New York, 1979.

Halleck, S. L. The initial interview with the offender. *Federal Probation*, 25:23–27, 1961.

Kaplan, H. I., and Saddock, B. J. The psychiatric report. In *Comprehensive textbook of psychiatry, Vol. 5*, H. I. Kaplan & B. J. Saddock (Eds). Williams & Wilkins, Baltimore, 1989.

Leon, R. L. *Psychiatric interviewing: A primer*. Elsevier-North Holland, New York, 1982.

Ludwig, A. *The importance of lying*. Charles C Thomas Press, Springfield, Ill., 1965.

MacKinnon, R. A., and Yudofsky, S. C. Outline of a psychiatric history and mental status examination. In *Textbook of psychiatry*, J. A. Talbott, R. E. Hales, and S. C. Yudofsky (Eds.). American Psychiatric Press, Washington, D.C., 1988.

Scheiber, S. L. Psychiatric interviewing, psychiatric history and the mental status examination. In *The American Psychiatric Association textbook of psychiatry*. American Psychiatric Press, Washington, D.C., 1988.

Stevenson, I. *The psychiatric examination*. Little, Brown, Boston, 1969.

Sullivan, H. S. *The psychiatric interview*. W. W. Norton, New York, 1954.

Werman, D. S. *The practice of supportive psychotherapy*. Brunner/Mazel, New York, 1987.

Whitehorn, J. C. Guide to interviewing and clinical personality study. *Archives of Neurology and Psychiatry*, 52:197, 1944.

Yalom, I. D. *The theory and practice of group psychotherapy*. Basic Books, New York, 1970.

Yalom, I. D. *Existential psychotherapy*. Basic Books, New York, 1980.

CHAPTER THREE

Taking the History: Part I

This chapter focuses on the kind of material that should be obtained in a psychiatric history with commentary on the best ways of obtaining it.

HOW SHOULD THE INTERVIEW BE INITIATED?

There is no uniform approach to beginning a psychiatric interview. The only rule of thumb is that physicians should begin by introducing themselves and saying something about their status, for example, "I am a medical student," or "I am the attending physician." This should be followed by a statement of what the physician will actually be doing (simply interviewing or conducting a physical examination as well), and how long it will probably take.

It is essential for patients to have a rough idea of the length of each interview, so that they can pace themselves and plan the rest of their day. Whenever possible, hospitalized patients should be given advanced notice of approximately when the interview will take place. When the physician is erratic and just "drops by," patients may be impressed by how busy the doctor is, but they are also insensitively reminded of their own powerless status. Patients are more cooperative when interviews are scheduled.

Once the essential courtesies are taken care of, there are three main opening gambits. First, the physician may try to ascertain the patient's chief complaint by asking questions such as "What brings you here?" or "How can I help you?" or "What is the main thing that is bothering you?" Second, the physician may wish to begin by inquiring about demographic data such as the patient's age, occupation, marital status, and residence. Third, the physician may wish to tell the patient a little bit more about himself or herself by elaborating on his or her level of responsibility for the patient's care, the kind of work he or she usually does, and how long he or she has been doing it. Although there are certain circumstances in which one or another approach is preferable, for most patients any of these opening gambits is acceptable.

Perhaps the majority of patients respond best to a straightforward inquiry about what is troubling them. This is especially true of voluntary patients who may be eager to seek help and want to get right to the business of telling their story. When the clinician has prior knowledge of why the patient has sought help through hospital records or through communications from whoever has arranged for the first meeting, this straightforward approach may have to be modified. In this situation, the patient is likely to know or expect that the physician knows something of his or her problems. A standard inquiry about what the complaint is may seem redundant or may cause the patient to fear that the physician has been too lazy or indifferent to learn about it. The physician who has prior knowledge of the reasons for referral may begin by saying to the patient, "I know a little bit about why you are here, but it would help if you could begin by telling me about it in your own words." Or the physician may summarize what is known about the patient's problem and combine a comment and a question, such as "I understand that you've had fears about leaving your house for two months now. Can you tell me more about this problem?"

If the physician knows that the patient is hospitalized involuntarily or is coming to an outpatient visit under the duress of his or her family or the law, a straightforward inquiry may also elicit annoyed or defensive responses in the patient. Too commonly, the committed patient responds to the question "What brought you here?" with "The police" or "An ambulance"; or to the question "Why are you here?" with "I don't know"; or to the question "How can I help you?" with "I don't need help. It's my wife who is crazy." If the physician knows that the patient is to be evaluated for commitment or is already hospitalized involuntarily, it is better to acknowledge this awareness by stating, "I know you are here against your will" and by asking a different type of question, such as "What is your understanding of how this situation came about?" This approach allows patients to maintain the stance that they are not sick or do not want help (both positions may be true) and to present their version of how their commitment came about. If the physician knows that the patient has been coerced into an outpatient visit, it may be useful for the physician to convey his or her awareness of the facts and to state, "I know you have expressed some reluctance to come here, but it is possible that you do need help, and I wonder if you can tell me if you have any problems." Or the physician may ask, "How did it happen that you came to see me under duress?"

The demographic approach may be most useful when the physician senses or knows from referral sources that the patient is extremely tense or agitated and needs to be put at ease. Here, it is important that the patient be able to respond coherently and successfully to the physician's initial inquiries. A general question such as "How can I help you?" may be perceived by an agitated patient as overwhelmingly complex. A better approach may be to ask initial questions that the patient is almost certain to answer correctly. A physician may say, "I am Dr. Jones, the chief resident in this ward. I'll be talking with you for the next hour in order to try to understand your problems. I'd like to begin by getting some information about you." Inquiries can then be made about various relatively neutral facts, such as the patient's place of residence, age, marital status, or occupation.

The evaluator's option of beginning the interview by talking about himself or herself may seem inefficient with regard to time and also too "folksy," but it can be very effective in encouraging communication by those who resent being in the role of a patient. When physicians tell patients a little bit about themselves, they create a more egalitarian relationship. They may also "disarm" the manipulative patient who is anticipating an authoritarian approach and is well prepared to resist it. When physicians sense or know that they are dealing with a patient with a serious personality problem, an opening such as the following may be useful: "Hi, I'm Dr. Smith, the attending physician on this ward. I'm going to try to evaluate your problem today by talking to you for the next hour, and I may be asking you a whole lot of questions. Before I begin, you may want to know something about me. I've been the attending physician here for about five years, and I've practiced psychiatry for about fifteen years. I'm originally from down south but now feel that this state is my home. I consider myself a general psychiatrist and try to see all kinds of patients and use all kinds of treatment. Now perhaps you can tell me a little bit about yourself." This technique is most comfortably used by experienced clinicians, who are comfortable in reverting from a folksy to a more businesslike relationship when this becomes necessary.

In some instances, the opening remarks of the physician must be preceded by a statement of the purpose of the interview and the extent to which it is confidential. Every patient has a right to be informed about the extent of confidentiality as soon as possible during the interview; at the same time, it is usually clumsy and unnatural to present this information when the patient and the doctor are first getting acquainted. Patients who come for help may simply not be interested in hearing about such issues before they even present their problems, and they may worry about the insensitivity of the physician who initiates an interview with a ritualistic explanation. It is quite another matter when the psychiatrist evaluates the patient for an agency. Here, the need for fairness may put limits on an unbridled quest for information. Patients who are being evaluated for agencies need to be told at the beginning of the interview why they are being evaluated, what kinds of issues the interviewer will be trying to evaluate, and exactly who will have access to the physician's report.

HOW DOES THE PHYSICIAN
FLESH OUT THE CHIEF COMPLAINT?

Some psychiatric patients give a direct and explicit response to questions such as "What can I help you with?" or "What's bothering you?" They may complain of personal experiences or behaviors that are troubling to themselves or others. Examples of direct complaints are "I'm depressed," "I'm too nervous to work," "I can't sleep," "I drink too much," "I can't think straight," "I have been thinking of killing myself," "I keep messing up my relationships," or "I keep writing bad checks."

Perhaps a larger group of patients voice a complaint that is vague or nonexplicit. Some examples of nonexplicit opening responses are "Something bad is happening to me," "I have this vague sense of impending doom," "I'm just not happy," "I don't think other people like me," "I'm really not much good at anything," or "I just can't cope."

A third group of patients come up with a traditional medical complaint even though they are aware of the fact that they are being seen for psychiatric evaluation. Examples of the chief complaints of this group of patients are "I suffer from backaches," "I have trouble breathing," "I'm sure I have cancer," "I'm tired all the time," "I'm nauseous all the time," or "I have bad nerves."

A fourth group of patients may not be able to enunciate a complaint. It is not uncommon for such patients to say, "I don't know what's wrong," "You have to tell me what's wrong," "I don't know why I came here," or "I just can't tell you about it."

Finally, there are patients who respond to inquiries regarding the chief complaint with replies that suggest severe psychopathology, such as "There is nothing wrong with me. It's just that the postal service is trying to kill me," "This computer they put in my stomach keeps telling me I'm going to die," "I've been impregnated by the devil," or "Why are you asking me about this? Are you from the CIA, too?" Non sequiturs or unintelligible or tangential responses may also be offered by the patient, and they, of course, suggest severe pathology.

In dealing with any of the above variety of "chief complaints," the examiner's task is to use the patient's initial response as a vehicle for obtaining a substantive and realistic picture of the patient's problems. The nature of the chief complaint, however, may dictate the exact approach that the clinician will take in fleshing out these details.

DEALING WITH DIRECT AND EXPLICIT CHIEF COMPLAINTS

When the patient comes in with an explicit chief complaint, such as "I'm depressed," an emphatic silence or a "tell me more" response on the part of the evaluator will usually elicit more details about the patient's distress. If this doesn't work, a variety of routine questions about the patient's experience can be asked; these relate to the frequency, length, or severity of the symptoms; what makes them better or worse; and what other symptoms are associated with them. This approach is used in all branches of medicine, but in psychiatry, something more is required. The examiner must try to determine what the patient means when he or she says, "I am depressed"; that is, the clinician must try to identify as precisely as possible the exact nature of the patient's experience. It is almost never safe to assume that the patients who say they are depressed really are. Such patients may be labeling perceptions of anxiety, confusion, anger, or guilt as depression, or they may be trying to put a conventional label on feelings too strange for them to identify. Or they may be trying to use the complaint of depression to gain access to the sick role.

Patients who report symptoms of depression must be told, "Depression often feels different to different people" and then asked, "What does it feel like for you?" This can be followed by questions that elaborate on all of the thoughts, feelings, and behaviors associated with these patients' perception of being depressed. Similar considerations apply to any chief complaint that refers to the patient's private experiences of distorted perceptions, unpleasant affects, or cognitive disturbances (such as forgetfulness or inability to concentrate). Intensive questioning about inner experience is the only means of obtaining an accurate picture of most major aspects of the patient's symptomatology. It also allows the clinician to understand what is happening to the patient and eventually to communicate that understanding to the patient.

The behavioral manifestations of troubling perceptual, emotional, or cognitive experiences should also be investigated. Once patients have explained the nature of their experiences to the best of their current abilities, they can be asked, "How does this feeling of depression affect your relations with people and your work?" or "What kinds of activities do your anxiety attacks prevent you from doing?" or "What do you do when you sense you're forgetting things or losing your train of thought?" In this type of questioning, the evaluator's focus is on relating patients' perceptions of distress to their social and occupational functioning. In moving from experiential to behavioral manifestations of the patient's illness, the evaluator learns a great deal about the severity of the patient's difficulty and about the extent to which the patient has been able to cope with her or his suffering. There may, of course, be inac-

curacies in the way patients depict their inner disturbances as influencing their behavior. Patients may minimize behavioral changes ("I don't
really drink very much when I'm nervous") or may exaggerate them
("I'm failing at my job. Everyone can tell I'm depressed because my
work has been so bad"). Wherever possible, the patient's perception of
disability must be checked against more objective information provided
by those who know the patient well.

When the chief complaint is manifested in behavior (complaints
such as "I keep getting into trouble all the time" or "I lose my temper too
much"), the evaluator must take a somewhat different approach. Here,
the behavioral symptom should be meticulously defined. Patients must
be asked to be as precise as possible in describing the exact nature of the
behavior that is causing difficulty. Once the clinician has a clear picture
of what behavior is troubling the patient, inquiries should be made
about its frequency and severity. The physician then explores whether
any events consistently precede or follow the behavioral symptom.
Here, the clinician is trying to determine whether certain stimuli regularly elicit the behavior, and whether certain consequences regularly
reinforce it. Once these data are collected, the clinician does almost the
reverse of what is done when the patient's complaint is manifested by a
disturbance of inner experience (when the inquiry is about how experience influences behavior); now, the physician asks about what thoughts
and feelings are associated with the troubling behavior. Questions such
as "What do you think about before, at the time of, and after you make
an obscene phone call?" or "What kinds of feelings do you experience
before, at the time of, and after your insult your wife?" help the evaluator
learn about distressing or deviant inner experiences that the patient may
never have otherwise volunteered. Such knowledge may be very critical
in treatment, because if the inner experience can be changed, the distressing behavior may be modified.

DEALING WITH NONEXPLICIT COMPLAINTS

Patients with nonexplicit complaints convey a sense of their distress
or disability to the physician in an imprecise manner. There are many
reasons for this kind of initial communication. These patients may be
truly unable to identify their feelings or to describe them (using such
terms as *depression, anxiety, anger,* or *apathy*) in a way that would be
recognizable to the physician. Or their problems with thinking may
have reached a level of severity that makes it difficult for them actually to
describe their experiences. Behavioral symptoms may be presented
vaguely when patients lack a complete awareness of the fact that things
are not going well in their personal relationships or their work.

There is no particular type of patient who presents with nonexplicit complaints. This group includes many with common psychiatric disorders (who may use nonexplicit complaints because they are poor observers or communicators of their feelings and conduct) but may also include patients with personality disorders, who are generally somewhat evasive, or people who have recently experienced some type of crisis that has threatened their sense of safety, security, and physical health.

With this group of patients, the physician begins by following up on the chief complaint, however vague it might be. If the patient says, "I'm just unhappy and don't know why," the clinician must try to identify what unhappiness feels like for that person and what other kinds of experiences are associated with it. Patients will seek to relate this kind of symptomatology to external events with statements such as "I'm under a lot of stress" (and this may be useful), but the physician should first be concerned with what the patient is actually experiencing. Questions such as "What does it feel like when you're unhappy?" and "How does your unhappiness show itself to others?" are helpful.

The physician's evaluative task will be facilitated if the patients can eventually describe their symptoms in terms that fall within the physician's range of experience. It is much easier for the physician to understand the patient who describes symptoms of depression than the patient who says, "I just feel strange." Physicians try to help patients put their symptoms into a more familiar context. They do this by inquiring about the possible existence of a commonly recurring group of disturbances of thought, feeling, and behavior ("Have you had trouble concentrating lately?" or "Do you ever feel like crying?" or "Are you irritable with your family?").

It is important that the patient not feel pressured to pigeon-hole his or her complaints in a category in which they do not fit. Sometimes, patients cannot relate their sense of "dis-ease" to any commonly understandable symptomatology. The physician should then try to avoid labeling the patient's symptoms and should continue the process of history taking in the hopes that, as other historical data are obtained, the patient's vague complaints will become more understandable. If, on the other hand, patients can genuinely translate their vague complaints into more explicit symptoms, these can be fleshed out just as any other explicit complaint can.

DEALING WITH TRADITIONAL MEDICAL COMPLAINTS

Most patients perceive their distress or disability as a medical disorder and initially seek out their customary (nonpsychiatric) physician. It is only as their medical evaluation fails to discover pathophysiological explanations for their symptoms that they are told that they may need psychiatric evaluation. Often, this news is both unwelcome and unacceptable. Referral to a psychiatrist may elicit fears of stigmatization or concerns that others will find them responsible for having created their own symptoms. These patients may be strongly committed to the idea that they have a bodily affliction, as yet undiagnosed by physicians, and that the only thing that will help them is an intervention that will cure it or simply remove it. They may not view themselves as active agents in their own treatment and may have great difficulty in understanding how their private experience, their behavior, or their environment may have contributed to their symptomatology.

Such patients are affronted by psychiatrists who do not take the medical aspects of their symptomatology seriously. The correct way for the psychiatrist to deal with patients who present with medical complaints is to begin by taking a medical history. If patients complain of pain, fatigue, or loss of appetite, these symptoms must be evaluated as they would be in any medical work-up. This procedure not only reassures these patients that they are being taken seriously and are not being labeled or stigmatized but also provides an additional review of earlier medical evaluations. It is entirely possible (and by no means uncommon) that a nonpsychiatric cause of the patient's difficulty has indeed been overlooked by other doctors.

As the patient's symptomatology is being investigated, the examiner can gradually shift over to more "psychiatric" questions, such as "How do you feel when people don't take your pain seriously?" or "Does all of this suffering depress you?" or "What do you think about when the pain is really bad?" or "What happens when you try to force yourself to do things in spite of the fatigue?" Once this type of questioning is begun, most patients are willing to shift to discussing problems they may have with thinking or feeling and how their symptoms have restricted their lives. As more traditional psychiatric symptoms are elucidated, they can be investigated in detail. It is useful, however, for the clinician to remind the patient periodically that the initial medical complaint has not been forgotten.

It is especially important that the psychiatric physician take a great deal of time in developing information about how any medical complaint has influenced the rest of the patient's life. This is the kind of information that other medical specialists may have glossed over, but it is obviously very important to the patient. Ultimately, it may provide many clues to what type of interventions will make the patient's life more comfortable. One variable that is especially critical in the lives of patients with chronic pain or with any other chronic medical symptom that appears to have no organic basis is litigation. This is particularly true if the onset of the symptom was due to an accident or was work-related. In my experience, over 80 percent of patients seen in pain clinics are in some type of litigation. It is important to know if patients are in litigation because this process does influence their attitude toward their illness, their treatment, and their recovery. A useful way to find out about litigation is to ask, after the history of the symptoms has been described, "With all the expenses you have incurred and all the suffering you have experienced with this pain, I wonder if you've tried any legal means of being compensated" This type of inquiry is not likely to encourage litigation, as most of these patients have already thought about it or are already in it. The inquiry may make it easier, however, for patients to talk about the litigation.

Beginning psychiatrists are often puzzled about how to respond to the patient who complains of "nerves." Such a complaint initially suggests a sophisticated patient who accepts the idea of having a psychiatric illness, and who may be an active participant in the process of treating it. Actually, the physician who takes the time to find out what the patient means by "nerves" usually discovers that the patient views "nerves" as an organic affliction of the central or peripheral nervous system. Such a patient may be reluctant to talk about inner experiences or behavior. The physician should deal with this kind of patient in the same way as with any patients who believe that their problems are nonpsychiatric illnesses.

DEALING WITH UNFORMULATED COMPLAINTS

Some patients may be aware that they are distressed or disabled but lack the ability either to identify the locus of their suffering or to communicate the nature of their difficulty to the physician. Occasionally, such patients are discovered to have a formal thought disorder or an expressive aphasia. More often, however, they simply are poor observers of themselves or poor communicators. With these patients, the physician must work hard. If the patient presents the message "I don't know what's wrong or why I came here, but I need help," the physician may want to reply, "It's often confusing to try to tell your problem to another person. Why don't you think about it for a moment or talk about something that you feel may be important for me to know." If the patient is still having difficulty, the focus can be shifted away from the chief complaint, and more time can be spent collecting historical data. Usually, the patient's recent history will provide clues to the symptomatology. Later, the physician can gently remind the patient that he or she did make the appointment or that someone else was concerned enough to make it and can ask, "What were you or others thinking about when you sought or were brought for psychiatric help?" If this question, too, fails, the physician can, in effect, conduct a "psychiatric review of symptoms" by naming a number of psychiatric symptoms and asking the patient if he or she has ever experienced them. This combination of techniques will eventually give the doctor some idea of why the patient has sought help.

A certain number of patients fail to reveal symptoms. They may do so for manipulative purposes or because they may be too embarrassed to describe what is troubling them. If the physician believes that either of these factors is operating, it may be useful temporarily to avoid elucidating the chief complaint and to inquire about past history and current life situation. A review of systems can then be made. With this kind of patient, however, it is unwise to let the initial interview end without making a rather forceful effort to obtain more information. It is always possible that the material the patient is withholding involves severe pathology or suicidal or homicidal intent. Even if the withheld material is more benign, the patient is likely to feel neglected or to be unimpressed by a doctor who has managed to get through the initial interview without making vigorous efforts to uncover it.

DEALING WITH INAPPROPRIATE COMPLAINTS

When a patient evaluated for involuntarily commitment is asked, "What's wrong?" or "How can I help?" a common response is "There's nothing wrong with me. If you want to help me, just get me out of here." There is always, of course, a possibility that the patient is right, and the physician must always be open to accepting this possibility. The best response to this kind of patient stance is "I really don't know if you have a mental illness or not, but somebody did think that you did, and perhaps we can explore what happened." The details of the process that resulted in the patient's proposed commitment or hospitalization can then be reviewed. Such a review usually allows the clinician to arrive at one of three conclusions: (1) the patient is clearly disturbed; (2) the patient is probably mentally ill but is presenting a distorted picture of the process that led to his or her possible commitment or hospitalization in an effort to avoid discussing the seriousness of the illness; or (3) the patient is not mentally ill and was incorrectly sent for evaluation or was even incorrectly hospitalized. The decision about which of the latter two conclusions may be correct takes time to make; often, it is not clarified until other aspects of the patient's history and mental status are explored or until objective data are available. If the clinician is concerned that a patient is distorting the reasons for the commitment or involuntary hospitalization, it may be best to leave the discussion of these issues for the moment and make inquiries about other possible symptoms or to go on to other aspects of the evaluation. Continuing the evaluation is also likely to help the clinician learn if the patient is, indeed, not mentally ill and should be discharged.

If patients respond to the physician's initial inquiries with what appear to be paranoid responses and are willing to talk about delusional ideas, it is useful to let them go on for a while. It may also be helpful to test the refractoriness of the delusional system to corrective input by giving such patients a chance to reconsider the basis on which it is maintained. If a patient insists that he is feeling sick because his wife is poisoning his food, he can be asked questions such as "What are your reasons for thinking that?" or "Why would she want to do that?" These questions help the patient reconsider the accuracy of his beliefs. If the patient responds with statements such as "I know I'm being poisoned because my food tastes strange" or "She wants me dead so that she can marry Ronald Reagan," it is useful to ask if there are other alternative explanations for these phenomena. Questions such as "Are there other possible explanations for the changes you perceive in your taste?" or "What are the reasons you believe your wife wants to marry the ex-president?" may provide a clearer picture of the patient's thinking. As the patient is required to consider his beliefs from a more conventional or logical perspective, he may indicate some doubt about their absolute validity. If the indication of doubt is an honest response, it suggests that the delusional system may not be immutable. If the response is simulated, there is reason to believe at least that the patient is sufficiently perceptive to be aware that his ideas may strike others as "crazy." The patient may, of course, continue to insist on the validity of his delusions, and this insistence tells the clinician that the patient's thinking and perception are severely disturbed.

It is difficult to conduct the above kind of dialogue with a patient who is agitated as well as paranoid. Gentle challenging of the patient's delusional belief is a technique best used with relatively calm patients. It also helps for the clinician to be open to the possibility that the patient's seemingly bizarre beliefs are true. Unless the patient's beliefs are patently bizarre or impossible (for example, "Fidel Castro is speeding up my aging process by bombarding me with gamma rays from Mars"), the clinician's unbiased effort to look at the evidence that the patient uses to sustain his or her beliefs will be perceived by the patient as supportive.

Some patients respond to the evaluator's initial request for information with non sequiturs or with tangential speech (these terms will be defined in the section on the mental status examination; for our purposes here, they refer to speech that appears illogical or not understandable). Such responses suggest serious disorders of psychotic proportion, sometimes based on demonstrable cerebral dysfunction. The evaluator should allow this kind of response to continue only long enough to familiarize herself or himself with the degree of the patient's pathology. Once the clinician has some idea of the nature of the patient's language disorder, it is useful to try to help the patient look more normal by shifting to the simplest type of questions, such as "How old are you?" and "Where do you live?" and "Are you married?" Some patients will become much more logical and understandable as their initial anxiety recedes. Others, generally those with organic brain disorders, may be unable to respond appropriately to even the simplest questions. Under such circumstances, the history must, of course, be obtained from other sources.

HOW LONG SHOULD THE PATIENT BE ALLOWED TO CONTINUE TO DISCUSS COMPLAINTS WITHOUT BEING INTERRUPTED?

The answer to this question depends on the evaluator's judgment of the usefulness of the information being presented and on the time available for evaluation. There is some variation in the manner in which clinicians of different schools deal with this problem. Doctrinaire neuropsychiatrists find little value in letting patients use up interview time in telling their story and prefer a style of active questioning. Doctrinaire humanistic or psychodynamic psychiatrists may feel that the ideal interview is one in which the examiner rarely interrupts the patient.

The clinician's willingness to avoid interruption will of course be determined by the amount of time available. In the emergency room, interruptions may be necessary soon after the patient begins. When there is a full hour or more available, the approach recommended here is that, during the initial interview, as long as patients are presenting useful material, it is advisable that they not be interrupted for as long as five to twenty minutes. This advice holds even when the material is not being presented in the exact order that the evaluator might wish, and the patient is skipping from symptom description to past history without filling in many obvious gaps. It is undoubtedly difficult for the evaluator to keep track of information that spans the present and the past in what is not always a coherent story. The examiner will be tempted to interrupt, to check out dates, to ask about additional symptoms, or to note connections between environmental events and symptoms. Nevertheless, it is best for the examiner to try to remember the various issues that the patient brings up and to postpone fleshing them out until later. Questions are best asked only when there are natural pauses in the patient's conversation; even then, comments such as "Please continue" or "Tell me more" may be more useful than questions that lead to a change of subject. Some patients want to tell their story in detail and experience considerable relief once they have told it. These patients may view the physician's interruptions as rude or insensitive. The additional stress that the interviewer experiences in withholding questions is more than compensated for by the trust and comfort that such withholding may provide for the patient.

On the "live-patient" section of the American Board of Psychiatry and Neurology oral examination, the candidate is allowed only thirty minutes to evaluate the patient. This time limit is similar to that in the emergency room. Most board examiners have concluded that candidates do best when they allow coherent patients to talk with limited interruptions for as long as five minutes. The rest of the examination always goes better when candidates curtail their anxiety during the initial part of the interview and avoid unnecessary interruptions.

WHEN IS THE BEST TIME FOR THE EXAMINER TO INQUIRE ABOUT ADDITIONAL SYMPTOMATOLOGY RELATED TO THE CHIEF COMPLAINT?

Although the physician must learn to think about the parts of the medical evaluation (such as the chief complaint, the history of the present illness, the past history, the review of symptoms, the physical examination, and the mental status examination) in an orderly manner, patients are rarely able to provide information about themselves in the exact manner the clinician would prefer. Most of the time, the psychiatric exam is a more spontaneous process during which information about a specific subject may be obtained at almost any time in the course of the examination. Nor are there accepted rules for when certain information should be sought. The mental status examination, for example, may be formally done after the history is taken; on the other hand, many aspects of the patient's mental status, such as the patient's appearance, language, memory, intelligence, judgment, and mood, can be continuously assessed as the history is reviewed.

One decision that must be made in every psychiatric interview is when to inquire about symptoms that are likely to be associated with the patient's major complaints. As physicians gain expertise, they learn that symptoms are usually clustered together. The patient who complains of feeling sad may also have appetite loss, sleep disturbance, anhedonia, difficulty concentrating, suicidal thoughts, low self-esteem, or irrational feelings of guilt. Patients who complain of difficulty in thinking may also be experiencing delusional ideas or hallucinations. By eliciting the presence of certain concurrent signs and symptoms, the clinician gains further understanding of the patient and is in a better position to make a DSM-III-R diagnosis. There are several points in the evaluative process where such inquiries about the presence of associated symptoms can be made. Some possibilities are when the chief complaint is being elaborated, as the history of the present illness is taken, as the patient's current or past history is assessed, or during some parts of the mental status examination.

The style advocated here is to begin inquiring about associated symptoms after patients have had several minutes to tell their stories and as the chief complaint is being elaborated. It is quite appropriate to inquire about symptoms such as weight loss or sleep disturbance as the details of a complaint such as depression are being fleshed out. This is also an appropriate time to ask about suicidal thoughts. The clinician need not adhere to this approach rigidly. If patients seem to want to tell their stories and are providing relevant information, inquiries about associated symptomatology can be made at a later time. It does make sense, however, to find out about all of the patient's symptoms as soon as possible. Most patients, as they discuss their chief complaint, make natural pauses that allow the evaluator to ask questions about associated symptoms. Patients may feel some relief in talking about these symptoms. They are also more likely to feel confidence in a physician who asks questions that imply a knowledge of the variety of experiences that are troubling them. The physician's early knowledge of all of the patient's symptoms may allow him or her to make more useful inquiries in subsequent stages of the examination.

WHAT ARE SOME OF THE COMMON PITFALLS IN EVALUATING ASSOCIATED SYMPTOMATOLOGY?

Any symptom that is revealed through questioning, rather than spontaneously, must be evaluated with the same thoroughness as the chief complaint. This would seem to be an obvious imperative; however, it is sometimes ignored by clinicians who are in too much of a hurry to confirm a diagnosis. Beginning physicians are especially prone to perfunctory questioning with regard to symptoms associated with affective disorders. Once the patient complains of depression, it is tempting to run through a checklist of the symptoms associated with depression and quickly to accept the patient's affirmative response as evidence that the symptom is present. More thorough questioning may reveal that the patient's initial affirmative response is insufficient evidence that the clinical condition actually exists.

When the patient complains of depression, the physician must always ask whether the patient also experiences elevated or irritable moods. Simple "yes" responses to questions such as "Do you ever feel hyper?" or "Do you ever feel as if you have unlimited energy?" or "Do people ever notice that you're very irritable?" or "Do you ever impulsively go out on a buying spree?" however, do not confirm the presence of these moods and do not in themselves offer sufficient evidence for a diagnosis of bipolar illness. Most people have experienced periods of feeling "high" or irritable, and most people have been impulsive at some time. To conclude that the patient has the symptoms associated with a manic episode, the clinician must find evidence of prolonged periods (of at least several days) of increased activity, pressure to keep talking, racing thoughts, decreased need for sleep, distractibility, and reckless behavior. Such evidence must be complied by asking a large number of questions about (e.g., the severity, duration, and consequences of) hyperactive behavior or by the documentation of such behavior by other reliable observers.

Even relatively measurable symptoms, such as weight loss or sleep disturbance, can be incorrectly assumed to confirm the diagnosis of depression when they actually have unrelated causes. In these days of preoccupation with personal appearance, it is important to inquire about whether the patient's weight loss was related to purposeful dieting. Sleep disturbances may be chronic manifestations of primary insomnia. Or they may be related to changing sleeping conditions, new work schedules, the behavior of the patient's bed partner, or physical illnesses.

WHAT KINDS OF QUESTIONS ARE USEFUL IN DETERMINING THE PRESENCE OF ASSOCIATED SYMPTOMS THAT THE PATIENT MAY NOT WISH TO DISCUSS?

Two issues that patients are often reluctant to discuss are suicidal thoughts and certain aspects of psychotic experience, such as delusions and hallucinations. Although an exploration of these symptoms can be considered part of the patient's mental status examination, it is often logical to inquire about their presence early in the evaluation. It makes sense to inquire about patients' suicidal thoughts while they are discussing feelings of hopelessness and despair. Similarly, it is reasonable to inquire whether agitated, fearful patients who are having difficulty relating their story to the examiner are experiencing delusional ideas or hallucinations. Although it is sometimes necessary to postpone inquiries into these issues until greater rapport is established, there are many advantages to obtaining this information early in the interview process. Knowledge of suicidality or psychotic thinking may lead to changes of emphasis in history taking and in the mental status examination; this is particularly true when time is limited.

Many severely depressed patients are reluctant to talk about suicidal thoughts or plans because they are ashamed of them. Or they may fear involuntary hospitalization if their thoughts are revealed. Imminently suicidal patients may, of course, avoid the subject because they do not wish to be prevented from carrying out their self-destructive wishes. In dealing with the severely depressed patient, the physician has no alternative but to pursue questioning about suicidality, even if such inquiries are troubling to the patient. A useful way to introduce the issue is to ask, "Do things seem hopeless?" or "How do you think this will all come out?" If these questions do not elicit information about self-destructive tendencies, the patient may be asked about suicidal thoughts or intentions in a more direct manner. Questions such as "Do you think about suicide?" or "Have you felt so bad that you've had thoughts of hurting yourself in some way?" may be appropriate. These inquiries should be followed by questions that help ascertain the history of the patient's suicidal behavior and the depth of the patient's current suicidal intent. When the clinician suspects that the patient is extremely ashamed of suicidal thoughts, less direct questions can be asked, such as "Do things ever get so bad that you wish you could just get away from it all?" or "At your worse moments, do you ever think about hurting yourself?"

When patients report thinking about suicide, it is useful to ask them if they are planning to commit suicide. Those who are still ambivalent about destroying themselves and who are trying to control their suicidal impulses are likely to acknowledge their plans. Unfortunately, those who are bent on self-destruction will not. When a patient does acknowledge suicidal plans, it is useful to inquire about its details. Such knowledge may help the clinician to judge the probability that the plans will be carried out. The overall problems of assessing suicidal and homicidal potential are important enough so that they will be discussed further in subsequent chapters.

Some severely depressed patients, of course, are not suicidal, and their negative responses to inquiries about suicide must be accepted. Other patients who are potentially suicidal may deny their suicidality but usually provide some cues to the examiner that they are covering up their intent. Long pauses, a vague and elusive answer, or vehement denials following inquiries about suicidality may be indications that the patient is not responding truthfully.

Delusional ideas are most likely to be expressed by severely and, usually, chronically ill patients. An open discussion of delusional ideas may presently suggest that the patient has little doubt that they are true or is too disturbed to appreciate that others will view these ideas as bizarre or "crazy." Less disturbed patients may cover up very bizarre delusions for months or years. Not infrequently, the psychiatrist who examines a patient who has recently committed a violent act may discover that the patient has harbored delusional ideas involving the victim for many years and has never told anyone about them. It is important to learn about these ideas, not only to make a diagnosis, but in some cases to prevent the patient from committing other harmful or self-destructive acts.

The clinician should inquire about delusions when patients complain of repetitive problems with other people (particularly when others are blamed for their problems), when they show any hints of problems in thinking, or when they are severely depressed. Patients whose discussions of interpersonal problems are dominated by a sense that they are regularly taken advantage of by others can be asked, "Do you ever feel especially singled out as a target by others?" or "It sounds as if you've had a rough time—why do you suppose people treat you so badly?" or "Does it sometimes feel as if these people are making fun of you behind your back?" If suspicious patients then begin to discuss thoughts that appear to be delusional, they may be willing to discuss more bizarre ideas if asked questions such as "Can you tell me how they are doing this to you?" or "What kinds of things are they saying about you?" Patients who complain of trouble in organizing their thoughts and who are clearly agitated sometimes reveal delusional material if asked questions such as "How do you explain what's happening to you?" or "Do you ever ask yourself how this could have happened?" Depressed patients who have self-depreciatory delusions can be asked, "Do you find yourself imagining terrible things about yourself that you would ordinarily not thing about?" or "Do you ever think that you feel so bad because of something you've done?" Depressed patients may answer these questions with an affirmative response that, though pathological (related to markedly diminished self-esteem), is not necessarily delusional. These questions, however, allow the patient to voice troubling delusional ideas if they are present.

It takes considerable skill to time these kinds of questions so that they are appropriate to the material that the patient is discussing. Questions about delusions should be asked with a sense of caring and concern. If the patient then reveals delusional material, the examiner must indicate interest in exploring it further without conveying any sense of either agreement or skepticism. Although the clinician may acknowledge to delusional patients that their ideas are unusual, the clinician's stance should be that of an investigator whose main purpose is to understand how patients have come to develop their ideas, and how their belief systems are affecting them.

One of the commonest problems confronting beginners in evaluating psychiatric patients is learning how to ask about hallucinations. (A discussion of the varieties of false or distorted perceptions will follow in the chapter on the mental status examination.) Inquiries about this type of symptom are best made after patients have revealed something about the depth of their disturbance, either by their behavior in the interview or by the nature of their complaints. The patient who is repeatedly distracted during the interview or who occasionally shouts at an apparent image that is not there can be asked directly, "Are you hearing or seeing things that are disturbing you?" Patients with chronic psychotic illnesses can often be asked in so many words, "Do you hear voices?" These patients have usually encountered so many indirect ways of being asked about hallucinations that they are just as likely to respond to a direct as a "subtle" approach. Patients whose disturbances are more acute may be more responsive to less direct questions, such as "With all the difficulties you've had, have you also had any strange experiences lately?" or "Sometimes people who are as upset as you are are troubled by hearing or seeing things that others do not—has anything like that been happening to you?" or "When you feel really bad, do you sometimes hear, see, or feel unusual things?" If the patient responds affirmatively to any of these questions, detailed inquiries should be made about the exact nature of the patient's experience and the situations in which it occurs.

Another useful but time-consuming way of getting at delusional or hallucinatory material is to ask patients to describe what they did on the day of the examination or the day before, beginning with their getting up in the morning. Using this technique, the clinician does not accept general responses such as "I got up and had breakfast" but inquires in meticulous detail about all of the patient's activities, such as brushing teeth, shaving, cooking breakfast, getting dressed, and the content of meals. Patients who do not have psychotic illnesses may have some trouble remembering details, but they will be able to account for most of their time. Highly disturbed patients will reveal large gaps in the day that they cannot account for. This response may, of course, reflect a disturbance of memory. But it is also useful to inquire if the unaccounted-for time was spent in ritualistic behavior based on delusional ideas or perhaps in listening to and trying to deal with false stimuli.

WHAT INFORMATION SHOULD BE OBTAINED IN TAKING A HISTORY OF THE PRESENT ILLNESS?

The history of the present illness should elucidate the manner in which the patient's symptoms have developed; in particular, how they have influenced and been influenced by the environment from the time they first began. One immediate task that confronts the examiner is determining when the symptom or symptoms began. Some patients perceive their major symptomatology to have developed at some precise moment in time and claim to have been symptom-free before that. Others, particularly those with personality and character disorders, may trace the origin of the symptomatology back to their childhood. Most patients describe an insidious onset of symptomatology, that is, a course in which the initial symptoms were minor and not too troubling, but in which there has been a gradual escalation of distress or disability.

It is desirable to begin taking the history of the present illness by asking patients when their symptoms began. If they have trouble answering this question, they can be urged to think back to a time when they were symptom-free and to describe what has happened since then. A few patients may insist that they can never remember having been symptom-free. With these patients, the clinician may want to deviate from the usual format and begin inquiry about past history, including symptomatology during childhood. Most patients, however, date the onset of symptomatology to a few days, weeks, or months preceding the examination.

One of the important assessments that the clinician must make in taking the history of the present illness is whether the patient's symptoms have been progressing, remaining static, or, perhaps, decreasing. It is also useful to know which (if any) symptoms have been intermittent and which continuous. This information can be obtained by asking the patient directly about when each symptom developed and how it has varied up to the present. The clinician should also keep in mind the effect of the wear and tear that the symptoms have had on the family and other individuals in the patient's environment.

It is helpful for the clinician to pursue the question relentlessly: "Why has the patient decided to seek help now?" or "Why has the patient been coerced to seek help now?" Inquiries into the issue of "Why now?" often uncover the presence of a previously unrevealed symptom, a new environmental stress, or the collapse of some environmental support system. These questions may also reveal the limits of the patient's coping mechanisms. This information may provide the clinician with ideas about how the patient's coping mechanisms can be strengthened or the environment modified in a manner that will alleviate the patient's dysfunction or distress. It may also help the clinician evaluate the severity of the patient's condition and may provide some clues to the immediate causes of the patient's distress.

Taking a detailed history of the present illness affords patient and evaluator an opportunity to consider the relationship of life events and particularly stressors to the patient's illness. Very few psychiatric symptoms develop out of the blue. Most frequently, they appear to follow stressful events in the patient's life. The history of the present illness is, in part, an effort to develop an account of the manner in which symptoms appear to be caused or influenced by environmental stress, or how the symptoms themselves may have elicited environmental responses that are in turn stressful. It is not always clear whether stressful events are the major causes of the patient's illness or are merely precipitating factors that bring out the illness in vulnerable subjects. In some instances, of course, the stress may have occurred coincidentally at the time the symptoms developed and may be unrelated to the symptomatology. Most of the time, stressful events contribute in some measure to the patient's symptomatology. The evaluator's knowledge of the relationship between stress and symptomatology is also useful in prognostication (if the stressors are severe, the prognosis may be better) and treatment (the removal of a stress or the avoidance of a future similar stress may diminish symptomatology).

Patients generally have a difficult time reporting or discussing the history of their present illness on their own; they may need a good deal of assistance from the physician in communicating this information. Questions such as "What happened next?" and "How did you feel when she did that?" and "What did you first try to do to cope with your sense of failure?" must be constantly fed to the patient in order to flesh out the details of individual environmental interactions. In taking this part of the history, it may be necessary, at times, to interrupt the patient and make sure that the time sequences of events and symptomatology are accurate. All of this is hard work for both the patient and the evaluator, particularly when the patient has many symptoms, is evasive, or has difficulty focusing on detail. The task of developing a detailed history of the present illness is easier if the evaluator is prepared to inquire about a comprehensive list of stressors and has a framework for organizing his or her thinking about what factors have been important in the patient's interaction with the environment as the illness has developed.

WHAT KIND OF STRESSORS SHOULD THE EVALUATOR INQUIRE ABOUT, AND HOW ARE THESE BEST CONCEPTUALIZED?

If two individuals are exposed to the same event, one may experience it as stressful and the other may not. As a rule, the severity of the stress is evaluated in two ways, both objectively, as the majority of rational people would be likely to respond to it, and subjectively, as a particular patient would respond to it. Common experiences validated by research provide clinicians with an objective sense of the severity of a stress and its probable impact on most people. Clinicians must also be willing to consider the possibility that some people perceive seemingly minor events as very stressful. For some patients, events such as having to wait too long at a restaurant or being left off an invitation list to a wedding may elicit powerful emotional reactions. Hence, in considering the impact of psychosocial stressors, the clinician begins by asking, "How would most people respond to this event?" and then proceeds to ask, "How has this patient responded to this event?"

Some patients directly relate their difficulties to psychosocial stresses. Here, the physician's task is to define the exact nature of the stress and to determine how it has influenced the patient. Other patients do not believe that their symptoms are related to psychosocial stresses even when the relationships are rather obvious. With patients who tend to view their symptoms as developing out of the blue, it is useful to inquire about a short list of possible stressors that may have been associated with the illness. These are generally related to family, work, money, or health problems. Some patients have a great deal of difficulty in observing their environment and in noticing how common stressors may be influencing them. Unless asked directly, these patients may not reveal how they have been influenced by significant environmental events. The clinician, of course, must always consider the possibility that the patient's perceptions are correct and that psychosocial factors have little to do with the illness or, on the contrary, that the patient is sometimes incorrectly attributing symptoms to stress.

In inquiries about stress, the routine categories of common events that should be considered include marital, family, financial, and occupational difficulties; legal problems; and recent physical illness. Stress in these areas can be created by accidental events that are outside the individual's control; it can also be created by the patient's own behavior. (An example of an accidental stress is the illness of a spouse. An example of a stress created by the patient's own behavior is a spouse's asking for a divorce after the patient has been sexually unfaithful.) The clinician is also concerned with unusual and often severe stressors, such as natural disasters. Another event (or series of events) associated with stress involves moving into a new phase of development in one's life cycle. Here, the clinician must consider such transitional events as leaving home, starting college, marriage, childbirth, retirement, or aging. Often, the patient is unaware of or minimizes the impact of developmental stress. The clinician can inquire about this kind of stress when the history of the present illness is taken or later, when past history and, particularly, developmental aspects of the past history are reviewed.

With patients who relate their symptoms to specific stressors, it may be useful to elaborate on these as they are brought up and to postpone a general review of other possible stresses until later. With patients who are unaware of the impact of stress on their problems, it may be useful to make inquiries twice, once at the time that the history of the present illness is taken, and later when the past history is reviewed.

What the psychiatrist deals with here is the complex nature of individual and environmental interaction as it relates to a mental illness. One useful way of conceptualizing this relationship is to think first of how the illness developed before any symptoms were noted by others (the presymptomatic phase) and then to examine what happened after such communication took place (the symptomatic phase). In considering the presymptomatic phase, the clinician focuses primarily on the causal influence of environmental stress in evoking symptoms. In particular, one seeks to determine if the major stresses that appear to have influenced the symptomatology were accidental, were related to developmental change, or were in the main caused by the individual's own psychopathology or personality traits. Accidental or developmental stressors suggest a better prognosis and are usually treated with less complicated forms of intervention. If it appears that patients are bringing stress on themselves as a result of their maladaptive personality traits, treatment is likely to be more difficult and prolonged.

In considering the symptomatic phase, the evaluator is concerned about a variety of critical issues. First, it is important to know about previous efforts to treat the patient's symptoms. In settings where residents or medical students work, previously untreated patients are hard to find. It is useful to inquire about what "home remedies" these patients have used, what professionals they have consulted, and what kind of treatment they have received. The history of previous medication often provides information about the kind of diagnoses others have entertained. When time is limited, this may be a very critical piece of information. It can describe which medications have worked, and which have not. It may also alert the evaluator to look for the presence of deleterious side effects such as tardive dyskinesia associated with certain types of medication. The history of previous psychotherapeutic efforts is also helpful; one can learn how patients have viewed psychotherapy, whether they have benefited from it, and how they have related to therapists of different persuasion or style.

A second kind of inquiry into the symptomatic phase of the present illness relates to responses of the environment to the patient's symptomatology. When patients complain of anxiety or depression, talk incoherently, or behave inappropriately, they have an impact on the environment. Such behavior may elicit responses of fear or distrust in others. Significant individuals in patients' environments may avoid them. These reactions create new stresses for patients. Angry and paranoid patients may elicit angry responses from others; these, too, are likely to engender new stresses. On the other hand, symptoms can also elicit a tender or reinforcing response from others. Some patients quickly discover that they receive more attention and nurturance from others when they are sick than when they are well. When the environment responds by reinforcing symptomatology, the symptoms often become very difficult to treat. The patient may be unwilling to abandon the nurturant aspects of the sick role. In this situation, the patient must learn new ways of seeking attention and nurturance, or those involved with him or her may have to learn to be less reinforcing when the patient is symptomatic and more reinforcing when he or she is well.

Sometimes, the patient is a valuable reporter of the environment's response to his or her symptoms. The patient can be asked directly, "Do people get angry when you are irritable?" or "Have you noticed whether people are troubled by your high moods?" or "Is your husband kind to you when you are so down?" It is often necessary, however, to obtain more information about environmental responses from family members, who may be more objective.

WHAT ARE THE MAIN ISSUES TO BE EXPLORED IN TAKING A MEDICAL HISTORY?

The completion of the history of the present illness is appropriately followed by a review of the patient's past psychiatric and medical illnesses. There is a natural order to this sequence, as the patient's past illnesses may have an obvious relationship to the current disturbance. It is important to know early in the interview whether the patient is suffering from a recurrent disturbance, is manifesting an old illness in a new manner, or is developing a new illness. If the pattern is a recurring one, it is especially important to inquire about previous treatment in order to learn which interventions have been most or least helpful. Sometimes, the history provides cues that allow the evaluator to comfort the patient. Patients who have recovered from a previous depressive episode and who have been symptom-free for many months or years may be reassured by being reminded that they have recovered from psychiatric disability before and should be able to do so again.

The history of nonpsychiatric medical illness can be taken in a very straightforward manner, as indeed it is in other branches of medicine. The only difference is that the psychiatrist is somewhat more concerned about such issues as how patients view their past illnesses, how the illnesses have interfered with their usual activities, how the illnesses influenced the environment, and how they may have influenced the patients' development. This information can also be obtained in the process of taking the past developmental history. In that phase of history taking, patients may recall past physical illnesses that they had forgotten to mention earlier.

The psychiatrist is also concerned about current nonpsychiatric illnesses that may have either an indirect or direct relationship to the patient's psychiatric symptomatology. Concurrent physical illnesses may have no direct etiological relevance to the patient's psychiatric disorders, but they may impose an additional and powerful stress on the patient. Sometimes the coexisting physical disorder is one that makes the use of certain psychotropic drugs risky. The course of the physical disorder may also be negatively influenced by the psychiatric disorder. For all of these reasons, the psychiatrist needs to have a clear picture of the patient's physical health and must be aware of how physical problems are influencing and are being influenced by the patient's mental disorder.

It is also true that there may be detectable physical causes of any psychiatric symptom. Although I emphasized in Chapter One some of the important differences between psychiatric and nonpsychiatric disorders, the clinician can never ignore the similarities. Psychiatrists must think just the way all other doctors do. When they observe behavioral or experiential symptoms, whether mild anxiety, depression, or severe psychosis, they must try to discover the pathophysiological processes that create these disturbances. They need to consider the possibility that neurological, endocrine, metabolic, toxic, nutritional, infectious, autonomic, or neoplastic disorders are major or contributing causes of the patient's psychiatric symptomatology.

Even though the patient may have been medically "cleared" by other physicians, if much time has elapsed since such clearance was obtained or if the symptoms are severe or atypical, it is useful for the psychiatrist to do a medical history, a review of systems that focuses on current medical difficulties, and a family medical history. It is especially important to focus on past or present neurological, endocrine, renal, hepatic, cardiac, or pulmonary impairment and on the family history of underlying brain disease (for example, Alzheimer's) or inherited metabolic disease (for example, diabetes or pernicious anemia). With certain patients, a careful taking of the medical history may provide new information about the patient's psychiatric problem. A review of systems, for example, with the schizophrenic patient may uncover the presence of bizarre ideas or even illusions or hallucinations related to bodily functions.

HOW DOES THE CLINICIAN OBTAIN MORE OBJECTIVE DATA?

It is possible to obtain relatively objective data regarding the patient's history from two sources: written or telephone reports of other professionals who may recently have examined the patient and reports of relatives or friends (and occasionally police officers or strangers) who have knowledge of the patient's recent behavior. Not infrequently, the patient's difficulties are acute, and there have been no recent interactions with other professionals. Even when reports have been written, they are often unavailable to the evaluator. This is particularly true of patients seen in emergency rooms or walk-in clinics, where sometimes the best a clinician can hope for is a very brief written report from a mental health professional, a police officer, or an interested person who may have petitioned for the patient's commitment. As a rule, the relatives and friends of the patient are a better source of objective information. Often, they will accompany the patient to the emergency room or walk-in clinic. If the situation is less critical and they are not present, they may be willing to talk to the doctor by phone or to come in for an interview if requested.

The observations of those who are emotionally involved with the patient cannot, of course, be purely objective. Relatives and friends may misperceive the patient's behavior, or they may have their own reasons for describing it in a distorted manner. Nevertheless, they are usually a reliable source of information, particularly about how the patient has been behaving in the pre- and the symptomatic environments.

Accurate information about any aspect of the patient's history is always welcome. As a rule, however, inaccuracy or incompleteness of information related to the patient's past history (particularly, the remote past) does not carry with it an immediate risk of diagnostic error. The developmental, educational, vocational, familial, and marital history may help the clinician understand why patients have become disturbed and may provide clues to the best way to respond to their illnesses, but it does not tell the clinician much about what is currently wrong with the patient. Thus, there is little urgency in obtaining objective information about this aspect of the past history.

The clinician's need to know about the patient's behavior in the very recent past is much more urgent. As noted in Chapter One, psychiatric diagnosis is often based on accurate descriptions of the patient's behavior. Patients are not always the most reliable observers of their own behavior. It is also likely that their behavior during the interview may be quite different from their behavior in other environments. Without objective data, the clinician can easily over- or underestimate the severity of the patient's illness. One of the more critical concerns is that the clinician will underestimate the risk that the patient is suicidal or imminently violent.

After completing the aspects of evaluation described thus far (the chief complaint, a history of the present illness, and the previous medical history), the clinician will often wish to interrupt the direct part of the interview with the patient and seek more objective data. There are circumstances in which it is especially important that the psychiatrist look for other sources of information about the patient's behavior; these arise when the patient appears to be having difficulty communicating, to be withholding information, or to be untruthful. At this juncture, the clinician can ask for the patient's permission to interview whoever may have accompanied him or her to the evaluative session, or the clinician may seek the patient's permission to telephone an individual who is likely to have direct knowledge about the patient's recent difficulties. There are, of course, many occasions when patients are able to provide comprehensive information without the assistance of others and may not wish to have the physician discuss their problems with others. To the extent that the physician is comfortable about the reliability of the data received directly from the patient and believes that the patient is not seriously disturbed, he or she should honor such a request. If the patient appears to be severely troubled, however, it may be prudent for the clinician to interview a family member or a friend, even when the patient does not wish that he or she do so.

If there is a critical need for objective data, and if those who might be able to provide it are not available, the clinician may have to call them on the telephone. This type of situation occurs most commonly when patients are brought to the psychiatrist for evaluation for possible civil commitment. Here, patients may deny statements recorded on commitment documents, which attest to their alleged mental illness or dangerousness. In deciding whether to sustain the commitment, the physician is obviously assisted by data beyond what the patient is willing or able to provide.

Telephone interviewing of family, friends, or acquaintances, whether they are the ones who petitioned for commitment or not, is fraught with pitfalls. Unless the clinician is certain that the person called knows that the patient is being evaluated, the clinician's call (unless sanctioned by the patient) is a violation of the patient's confidentiality. It is also difficult to interview people over the telephone. Those interviewed may be reluctant to say very much to a strange doctor who calls them unexpectedly. If they happen to be petitioners, the fact that they did not call the doctor themselves and that they did not accompany the patient to the hospital or clinic may indicate that they have negative feelings toward the patient. Some who are called may have strong reservations about involuntary hospitalization and may minimize symptomatology. Others may have personal reasons for wanting to see the patient hospitalized and may exaggerate symptomatology.

In calling a stranger, the physician does best by explaining the situation to the person and then inquiring about facts relevant to the patient's mental illness. An introduction such as the following might be appropriate:

> "Hello, Mrs. Jones. I'm Dr. Peters, and I'm calling from University Hospital. Your brother Jim has been sent to the psychiatric emergency room here at

> University Hospital on commitment papers. The papers say that he has been making threats to his mother and you, but he denies that this is true. He does seem very agitated right now, and it is hard to evaluate what actually happened because nobody accompanied him to the emergency room. He was just brought here by the sheriff after the papers were served. I know that you may be very upset by what I have just told you, but I hope you can give me some information. He has given me permission to talk to you. Can you tell me, first of all, whether your brother has made threats against you? Then, I would like to ask you some more questions about the general state of his health and his recent behavior."

When relatives, friends, or acquaintances who can provide objective information are available in the clinic or the emergency room they can be interviewed privately, but there are some occasions when it is advantageous to have patients participate in a conjoint interview. The latter approach is likely to be indicated when patients are not overly disturbed, when they wish to be present, or when their relationship with the accompanying person or persons appears to be a critical factor in their disturbance. A conjoint interview has the advantage of letting the patient and the accompanying person or persons interact with one another and perhaps correct one another's information. It also gives the clinician an opportunity to observe how the patient interacts with significant others in his or her life.

Whether the accompanying person is seen with or without the patient present, it is useful to begin this aspect of the interview with a statement such as the following: "I have been asking Mr. Jones about his difficulties, and he has been describing them to me. So far I have learned the following. . . . " At this point, the clinician briefly summarizes what has been learned from interviewing the patient and says, "I wonder if you see things the same way or if you can add any information that will help me understand what is happening?"

It is generally reassuring when the accompanying person confirms the patient's version of the present illness and even adds a few details that the patient may not have noted or may have forgotten. The clinician may be somewhat less reassured when the accompanying person brings out information that the patient deleted or that may contradict what the patient said, but that the patient may in retrospect be willing to accept as accurate. Here, the clinician is wise to be concerned about the patient's reliability as a reporter but can usually (but certainly not always) assume that the accompanying person's version of the history is accurate.

More serious difficulties arise when the patient and the accompanying person provide contradictory information about what has been happening to the patient, and neither changes his or her story. When this happens, the accompanying person is usually describing—and the patient denying—highly deviant behavior such as excessive drinking, violence, or talk of suicide. Here, the clinician has a serious problem. If the behavior reported by either party is not severe enough to warrant hospitalization, the best thing that the clinician can do is simply to suspend judgment about what is actually wrong with the patient and to rely on more time and more evaluation to provide an answer. If the accompanying person reports behavior suggestive of severe mental illness or dangerousness, however, it is usually best to take a conservative approach and to hospitalize the patient. There will, of course, be times, when the patient appears to be more rational than the accompanying person, and the clinician will be concerned that the hospitalization is inappropriate. In my experience, however, efforts to "railroad" patients in the current era of intensive legal surveillance of the commitment process are extremely rare.

FOR FURTHER READING

Balint, M. *The doctor, his patient and the illness* (2nd ed.). International Universities Press, New York, 1972.

Hales, R. E., and Yudofsky, S. L. *Textbook of neuropsychiatry*. American Psychiatric Press, Washington, D.C., 1987.

Hall, R. C. W. (Ed.) *Psychiatric presentations of medical illnesses: Somatopsychic disorders*. S. P. Medical and Scientific Books, New York, 1980.

Henden, H. Psychodynamic motivational factors in suicide. *Psychiatric Quarterly, 23*:672–678, 1951.

Lazare, A. The psychiatric examination in the walk-in clinic: Hypothesis generation and hypothesis testing. *Archives of General Psychiatry, 30*:96–102, 1976.

Leon, R. L. *Psychiatric interviewing: A primer* (2nd ed.). Elsevier, New York, 1989.

Leon, R. L., Bowen, C. L., and Faber, R. N. The psychiatric interview, history and mental status examination. In *Comprehensive textbook of psychiatry*, Vol. 5. H. I. Kaplan and B. J. Sadock (Eds.). Williams & Wilkins, Baltimore, 1989.

Lewis, N. D. C. *Outline for psychiatric examination* (3rd ed.). State Department of Mental Hygiene, Albany, New York, 1943.

Masserman, J. H., and Schwab, J. J. *The psychiatric examination*. International Medical Books, New York, 1974.

Menninger, K. *The human mind*. Knopf, New York, 1945.

Miles, C. P. Conditions predisposing to suicide: A review. *Journal of Nervous and Mental Diseases, 164*:231–246, 1977.

Pasnau, R. O., and Fawzy, F. I. Stress and psychiatry. In *Comprehensive textbook of psychiatry*, Vol. 5. H. I. Kaplan and B. J. Sadock (Eds.). Williams & Wilkins, Baltimore, 1989.

Pokorny, A. Prediction of suicide in psychiatric patients. *Archives of General Psychiatry, 40*:249–257, 1983.

Pruyser, P. W. *The psychological examination: A guide for clinicians*. International Universities Press, New York, 1979.

Rane, R. A., and Arthur, R. J. Life change and illness studies: Past history and future directions. *Journal of Human Stress, 4*:3, 1978.

Reiser, D. E., and Schroder, A. *Patient interviewing: The human dimension*. Williams & Wilkins, Baltimore, 1980.

Resnick, H. *Suicidal behavior*. Little, Brown, Boston, 1968.

Rosen, V. H. The initial psychiatric interview and the principles of psychotherapy. *Journal of the American Psychoanalytic Association, 6*:154–167, 1958.

Rutter, M., and Cox, A. Psychiatric interviewing techniques. 1: Methods and measures. *British Journal of Psychiatry, 138*:273–282, 1981.

Scheiber, S. C. The psychiatric interview, psychiatric history and mental status examination. In *Textbook of psychiatry*. J. A. Talbott, R. E. Hales, and S. C. Yudofsky (Eds.). American Psychiatric Press, New York, 1988.

Stevenson, I. *Medical history taking*. Hoeber, New York, 1960.

Taylor, M. A. *The neuropsychiatric mental status examination*. Spectrum Publication Books, New York, 1981.

Waitzkin, H., and Stoeckle, J. D. The communication of information about illness. *Advances in Psychosomatic Medicine, 8*:180, 1972.

CHAPTER FOUR

Taking the History: Part II

The past history reveals a picture of the patient's life experiences and behaviors from birth to the present. Not all of this information is relevant to diagnosis. In fact, most DSM-III-R diagnoses can be made with only token recourse to past history. Nevertheless, the past experiences do have a major influence on the patient's current illness. Some experiences may be necessary or sufficient causes of current symptomatology. Other experiences foster the development of personality traits that influence the manner in which the patient deals with symptomatology and is influenced by treatment. At least some knowledge of the patient's past learning experiences is essential to the successful utilization of most forms of psychotherapy.

Some schools of psychiatry have believed that different symptom complexes (as revealed by the chief complaint and the history of the present illness) are associated with rather specific past learning experiences. Clinicians of these schools recommend that the evaluator pay special attention to particular aspects of the past history that are alleged to be most relevant to the current symptomatology. This approach is not recommended here. I am unconvinced that we know enough about etiology to relate specific past experience consistently to specific present symptomatology. There are some important exceptions. It does make sense, for example, for the clinician to search hard for history of childhood sexual or physical abuse in patients who appear to have serious personality disorders, who appear to have dissociative experiences or who are themselves abusive. Overall, however, history taking is best viewed as a systematic fishing expedition. The clinician focuses on as many aspects of the past history as time allows and keeps an open mind about which aspects of the past experience of patients may be exerting influence on their current symptomatology. In short, the clinician should not approach the patient with an excessive bias about which life events are most likely to be related to the patient's illness. To ensure thoroughness, the clinician should make at least some inquiries about patients' development as children; the influence of their family; their schooling; their work; their social activities, including sexuality; and their own marriage and parenting.

The family history is an important part of the past history. Sometimes, the family history is viewed, literally, as a history of the major life experience of the patient's family members, with particular reference to any mental illnesses they may have experienced. This, however, is only one aspect of the family history. The term may also refer to the manner in which family members have interacted with and influenced the patient. Many of the patient's more powerful learning experiences are engendered by such family interactions.

For both participants, reviewing the past and family histories is generally the easiest part of the psychiatric examination. Patients tend to be less stressed when talking about the past than when dealing with present difficulties. As noted in Chapter One, there really is no limit to the amount of material that can be elicited, for an examiner will find that any kind of information the patient reveals is likely to be of at least some value. If the patient is having difficulty communicating and the interview is not going well, or if the psychiatrist doesn't have any sense of what should be done next, a safe "fall-back" position is to take more history.

The psychiatrist may find that a patient is just as poor an informant about past history as he or she has been about the chief complaint and the history of the present illness. Interviews with family members may then be required to provide a more objective picture of the patient's past, particularly early childhood development. Insofar as they may provide more than one perspective on a particular historical event, conjoint family interviews may also be useful. This phase of searching for objective history can be conducted in a relatively leisurely manner.

HOW DOES THE PHYSICIAN MAKE THE TRANSITION FROM THE CHIEF COMPLAINT AND THE HISTORY OF THE PRESENT ILLNESS TO THE PAST HISTORY?

Although the past history is written or presented in an orderly manner (usually childhood history is presented first, followed by school, occupational, sexual, marital, and family history), the physician does not have to begin history taking by focusing on any specific area. It is likely that, in the course of presenting the chief complaint and the history of the present illness, the patient will allude to experiences involving family, schooling, work, or relationships with peers. The physician can begin past history taking by making inquiries about how these experiences have influenced the patient over time. If the patient's current illness is characterized by work-related difficulties, for example, there is a certain logic and naturalness about beginning past history taking with a review of the patient's employment history. If the patient complains of interpersonal difficulties, inquiries about past history can begin with questions about previous relationships, including those with other family members.

Another tactic that the clinician can use is to allow the patient to choose where to begin by offering an open-ended question such as "Now that I have a pretty good idea of what's troubling you, I'd like to learn more about you as a person. Can you tell me a little bit more about yourself?" Information can first be collected about whatever area the patient chooses to bring up, and the examiner can then comfortably move on to inquiring about another area.

The patient's discussion of his or her present or past illnesses may provide a natural link to the family history. It is always important to know if other family members have had difficulties similar to those of the patient. As these inquiries are made, additional questions can be asked about other illness experiences of family members. The physician will then want to know how these illnesses affected the family member, and if they influenced that person's relationship to the patient. As this discussion continues, it can gradually merge into a consideration of other aspects of the patient's interaction with that particular family member. Through this discussion of illness experiences, important aspects of the patient's developmental and family history should unfold.

Finally, even if no natural and comfortable bridges seem to develop, and if there is a painful silence after the patient has discussed the chief complaint and the history of the present illness, there is nothing wrong with the examiner's saying, "I'd like to learn a little bit more about your past. Can you tell me about your family? Your schooling? Your previous jobs? Your childhood?"

WHAT ARE THE MAIN ISSUES THAT THE PHYSICIAN LOOKS AT IN TAKING A PAST HISTORY?

In developing information about how the past history is relevant to the present symptomatology, it is useful for the clinician to make three general types of inquiries: (1) How did certain characteristics of the past environment adversely influence the patient? (2) How did certain characteristics of the patient interfere with his or her capacity to meet environmental expectations? And (3) how has the environment responded to the patient's deficiencies?

As noted in the previous chapter, many aspects of the environment that are likely to influence the patient adversely can be thought of as stresses. Some stresses, such as being subjected to child abuse or having a curable physical illness, have an immediate and direct influence on the patient. Other stresses are more chronic and insidious, such as those created by nonnurturing parents, poverty, or a meaningless job. Characteristics of patients that may interfere with their capacity to deal with the environment include learning difficulties, physical handicaps, shyness, limited intellectual abilities, addiction-proneness, violent proclivities, and other maladaptive personality traits. The environment's response to the patient's incapacities include variables such as rejection by family members, negative responses of school officials to a poor learner, and lack of sufficient social and occupational opportunities. These latter environmental responses, of course, constitute new stresses for the patient. The individual-environmental interactive processes in this situation may lead to a gradual escalation of symptomatology.

Obviously, the process of individual–environment interaction involves each variable's responding continuously to the other. In the midst of all of this, the clinician has to begin somewhere. The search for answers to the three questions listed above, insofar as it allows for the examination of observable and measurable parts of a very complex process, provides a mechanism for starting.

Before launching into taking the past history, the clinician should be reminded that, although much emphasis is usually put on stressful events, it is also important to note their absence. Positive reports to the effect that the patient was very much loved, develop normally, and did well with friends and at school should always be noted.

WHAT IS THE MOST PERTINENT INFORMATION THAT THE EVALUATOR CAN OBTAIN ABOUT THE PATIENT'S EARLY CHILDHOOD?

Some of the events that influence patients are present even before they are born. The mother's health during pregnancy is of special significance. Inquiries should be made about whether she used alcohol, tobacco, or any other drugs during her pregnancy. There are also social circumstances in the prenatal period that may put undue stress on the child from the day of birth. If the mother was unwed, separated from her husband, physically or mentally ill, or living in poverty, she may not have welcomed the birth of the patient or may have lacked the capacities to provide her child with adequate nurturance. Such circumstances do not inevitably lead to poor parenting, but they do increase the probability that it will occur. Ordinarily, the patient can provide little factual information about the presence of severe stress on the family in the prenatal period; this information must generally be confirmed by other observers.

Any handicap that children bring into the world will be a source of stress both for them and for those who take care of them. Perhaps, the most frequent handicap is prematurity. One of the most troubling aspects of prematurity is that the child is often separated from the mother during its first days of life. If bonding does not take place between mother and child early in the child's development, the child may be at risk of subsequent abuse from the parents. Physical handicaps, particularly if they interfere with the feeding process, tax the capacities of parents to provide nurturance; the presence of such difficulties may also influence the parent's subsequent relationship to the developing child. As a rule, the patient is aware of physical handicaps that were present at birth and can tell the physician about them. The manner in which the parents dealt with the child's handicap, however, is something that they alone are likely to know.

The clinician can learn about acute and time-limited stressors in early childhood by asking patients directly about accidents or illness to themselves or their parents at this time in their lives. Inquiries about nonsexual and sexual physical abuse must usually be made in a more delicate manner, and some hints for making this kind of inquiry are presented in a later section. The presence of chronic stress is revealed through questions that are part of the family history. Information about possible sources of stress, such as the marital situation of the patient's parents, their health, or their socioeconomic status, should be obtained for each developmental period that the clinician is investigating, as these variables change over time. The influence of any given stress will also have varied with the patient's stage of development. In investigating the first year of the patient's life, the clinician is especially interested in any adverse family circumstances, such as separation, divorce, parental illness, or poverty, that resulted in changes in the nurturing capacities of the child's primary caregivers.

Another important aspect of the patient's early development is the presence of siblings. The birth of younger siblings significantly dilutes the amount of nurturance that parents can provide the patient. Inquiries about the ages of siblings during the patient's earlier years should be noted, and efforts should be made to define sibling problems that were stressful.

Any severe illness (such as congenital heart disease or asthma) that the patient experienced in early life should be considered in terms of its impact on the patient and the environment. Illness is, of course, in itself a stressful experience, but the child–parent interaction that takes place in the course of dealing with the illness may be even more important.

Parents tend to treat a sick child differently, and if illness is life-threatening or chronic, some of the changes in their manner of parenting will have long-term effects. Not uncommonly, a sickly child may be viewed as needing more protection or attention. Parents may diminish their expectations of such a child's short- or long-term accomplishments. It is useful to inquire if patients recall or have been told about any severe illnesses in the first five years of their lives. Following this inquiry, they can be asked if their parents have ever said anything to them about how illness may have influenced their upbringing. Usually, this information is difficult to obtain without interviewing the family.

One disorder that is common and that significantly influences how the child behaves and how the parents respond to the child is attention-deficit hyperactivity disorder. This disorder begins before the age of seven and is characterized by peculiarities of motoric and attentive behavior that put an enormous stress on parents. Their responses to the child's distractibility and hyperactivity are also likely to stress the child.

Children vary in their rates of development; parents, in turn, vary in how they may define a particular child's development as delayed, and in how they respond to their perception of delay. The evaluator usually inquires about any problems that the patient was told about in regard to walking, talking, toilet training, playing with other children, or tolerating separation from the parents. If it turns out that the parents perceived the patient's development as abnormal, it is useful to try to find out how they felt that abnormality influenced the child and how they responded to the situation. Such information is also likely to be difficult to obtain without the assistance of the parents.

Ordinarily, the accuracy of the information obtained from history taking is variable, and information about early childhood is especially prone to distortion both by the patient and by those who raised him or her. People tend to recall their past in a manner that explains and justifies their past actions or current deficiencies. Often, this process involves a failure to remember some events, placing exaggerated importance on other events, or even a false reconstruction of past reality. Some psychiatrists are more troubled by their patient's inability to provide an accurate past history than they need to be. Our knowledge of how early experience affects subsequent symptomatology is not so precise that we can regularly relate specific events to specific symptoms. What the physician is looking for are patterns of maladaptive learning that are directly or indirectly related to current symptomatology, and that may be modifiable by treatment. These patterns are inferred by examining a number of variables, including the patient's current and past behavior, the patient's and the patient's caregivers' perception of the past, and the physician's factual knowledge of what actually happened in the past. It is, of course, desirable for the physician to have information that is as accurate as possible; this dictum pertains to all aspects of the patient, including early development. However, the physician should be able to use even a distorted historical presentation to infer the existence of maladaptive learning patterns.

The usefulness of imprecise or even inaccurate information about early childhood may be illustrated by considering a question that psychoanalytically oriented psychiatrists commonly ask patients: "What is your earliest memory?" The patient's responsive description of an event may be less than accurate for a variety of reasons. Still, it may reveal how the patient retrospectively views his or her childhood and may substantiate other inferences that the physician has drawn about the kinds of maladaptive learning experiences that are currently influencing the patient. Thus, a highly perfectionistic patient who always fears doing something wrong may come up with an earliest memory of vomiting on his new suit of clothes and being punished for it (a not uncommon type of earliest memory for this type of patient). This recollection, in turn, may cue the physician to look for other evidences that the patient was raised in an environment in which there were unusual demands for perfection. This knowledge would then set the stage for a better understanding of current symptomatology, opening the way to appropriate behavioral or psychotherapeutic intervention.

WHAT INFORMATION DOES THE PHYSICIAN SEEK ABOUT THE PATIENT'S DEVELOPMENT DURING THE MIDDLE YEARS OF CHILDHOOD (AGES FIVE TO TWELVE)?

Information about significantly stressful environmental events in middle childhood is pursued in the same manner as information about early childhood. The impact of stresses such as divorce in the family or the illness of a significant caregiver is, however, somewhat different for the older child (although there is no clear consensus about how it is different). The clinician will also wish to inquire into any health or adjustment problems that the patient experienced during this period. Some of these problems, such as nightmares, phobias, bed wetting, fire setting, or excessive masturbation, can be viewed as responses to a stressful environment. Insofar as parents and other caregivers must respond to these behaviors, they also influence the environment.

One of the unique developmental events in middle childhood is leaving the primary caregivers for a significant part of the day and going to school. Although the patient may have had experience with day schools and nurseries before age five, the beginning of grade school on a daily and more-or-less full-time basis constitutes a major challenge. It is something children must meet and master if they are eventually to adjust to our society successfully. Many emotional problems first emerge when children are asked to meet this developmental task, and it becomes a major challenge and a major stress if it is not met in a manner that others judge to be satisfactory. One of the commonest problems at this stage of development is school phobia. It is useful to inquire whether the patient ever had problems in getting to school or remaining in school and, moreover, if there were problems, how the parents dealt with them.

In addition to learning about evidence of school avoidance, the clinician will also be interested in the patient's school performance. One major issue here is the existence of learning problems related to specific developmental disorders. (These may involve reading, language expression, writing, or coordination.) Asking about school difficulties also provides a second opportunity to learn about attention-deficit hyperactivity problems. A child who is having difficulty learning in school because of hyperactivity or a developmental disorder may develop a diminished sense of self-esteem, may have difficulty relating to peers, or may be stigmatized by teachers and viewed as a nonrewarding or troublesome student. Failure to perform adequately in school may also lead to difficulties at home. Some parents may be especially indulgent to children who are having learning difficulties, whereas others treat them more harshly.

Information about the patient's learning capacities and the environment's response to any associated problems can be gained by direct inquiry. Straightforward questions such as "What was it like for you in grade school?" or "How did you do in school?" or "Did you have any trouble learning how to read or write or do arithmetic?" or "Did you have many discipline problems with your teachers?" are usually answered directly. In inquiring about the later grade-school years, the physician may wish to ask which subjects posed the most difficulty for the patient, and which were most rewarding. Responses to these questions give the physician some early clues to whether the patient's strengths and weaknesses lie in conceptual thinking, verbal and symbolic characterization, motor performance, spatial perception, or artistic creativity.

By the time the child enters grade school, certain patterns of socialization began to emerge. It is useful to inquire about friendships and relationships with peers during this time period. A lack of ability to make friends because of shyness, aggressivity, lack of attractiveness, or some handicap should be noted. Loneliness during this period may increase feelings of sadness, and these in turn may significantly influence school performance. Patterns of relatedness also begin to develop during this period. The clinician will want to learn whether the patient was able to sustain friendships on an egalitarian basis, or if there were early signs of exploitiveness, demandingness, manipulation, or ingratiation in interpersonal relationships.

It is useful to inquire about the patient's early relationships with teachers. Differences in the way the patient related to male and female teachers should be noted. Such information may confirm a pattern of relating to adults that parallels that of relating to parents and other authority figures. Teachers may also be a source of unusual stress in the patient's early life; on the other hand, they may sometimes provide nurturance or reinforcement that compensates for inadequate parenting.

The patient's early interest and level of success in sports and hobbies should be noted. In this regard, it is probably useful to try to determine the number of hours patients spent watching television during the formative years of their live. Sufficient scientific data are still unavailable concerning the long-term effects of devoting a large part of one's childhood to watching television. It is probably safe to assume, however, that an individual who has spent a very large part of his or her early life staring at a small picture tube has less vitality, creativity, and self-esteem than an individual who has used those same years for reading, participating in sports, or cultivating hobbies.

The review of the events of middle childhood affords the most appropriate opportunity to inquire about whether the patient was physically or sexually abused as a child, although this is not the only possible point of inquiry. Other suitable opportunities for this kind of inquiry occur when the history of early childhood, past sexual experiences, or problems experienced by the parents are investigated. Some patients volunteer their history of past abuse, others talk about it only if asked, and still others talk about it only if approached in a very gingerly and tentative fashion. Finally, there are many patients who recall experiences of abuse, but who nevertheless deny them (although this response is becoming less frequent as more information about its prevalence becomes available to the public).

When evaluating patients whose parents were involved in antisocial conduct or who regularly abused alcohol or other drugs, the physician should suspect that the patient was abused as well. A similar assumption can be made if the patient's presenting symptoms are suggestive of personality disorder characterized by repeated self-harmful behavior, low self-esteem, and being either exploited or exploitive in interpersonal relationships. Patients whose symptoms are characterized by a frequent use of dissociative defenses and particularly those who have symptoms characteristic of multiple personality disorder are also likely to have been abused as children.

The physician can usually make some determination about whether patients will respond to direct questioning about child abuse by noting how frank they have been in discussing negative aspects of their past or of their family. If patients paint a "rosy" picture of the past and the physician doubts that it is accurate, indirect questioning is preferable. On the other hand, if patients seem willing to discuss freely the negative aspects of their past and their family, questions about abuse can be posed more directly. It should be noted that some patients who have been subjected to violent discipline respond negatively to questions regarding abuse, even when they wish to be truthful. These patients may view extreme forms of corporal punishment as part of the cultural norm; they will assert that it is good for them, and they will not suspect that the experience may have had harmful consequences.

One indirect way of uncovering a history of abuse is to inquire about patterns of discipline during early and middle childhood. The frequency and severity of corporal punishment can be noted. It is also important to inquire about the degree to which physical punishment was associated with experiences of humiliation. Public punishment (with siblings or friends observing) or punishment while partially or fully undressed may be especially traumatic. The question of when physical punishment should be viewed as abusive is, of course, related to cultural perspectives. The important issue here is how patients felt about the kind of punishment received and how it might be influencing their present symptomatology.

If either parent abused alcohol or other drugs, it is sometimes useful to make inquiries such as "How did your father behave when he was drunk?" or "Was he ever physically abusive to your mother?" or "Did he ever physically abuse you while intoxicated?" or "How was this done?"

In considering the relationship of fathers, stepfathers, or other male caretaking figures to daughters, it is a relatively easy step to move from inquiries about physical abuse to questions of sexual abuse. Inquiries such as "When your stepfather was drunk, did he ever try to have any kind of sexual contact with you?" are appropriate. If the patient responds affirmatively, she can be asked, "What did he try to do?" The patient can then be asked about her response to this kind of victimization. The physician should not be surprised if the patient has little to say about an experience of sexual abuse. Many patients have great difficulty remembering or describing their emotional response to sexual molestation.

Sexual molestation in our society appears to be so common (38 percent of girls and 9 percent of boys) that inquiries about it should be a routine part of history taking. The physician must be concerned with molestation not only by family members but also by other adults in the community as well. One useful way of obtaining this kind of information is simply to state, "We now know that sexual molestation is a very common experience in our society, and that it often has a negative impact on an individual's mental health and development. Can you recall any experiences during your childhood in which any adult tried to touch you or to relate to you in an erotic way?"

There is convincing evidence that the majority of children coerced into sexual activity (particularly if the coercion is associated with the penetration of body orifices) experience subsequent emotional disturbance. At the same time, it is very difficult to decide how traumatic less violent erotic experiences with adults have actually been. Some sexual encounters with adults are not painful to the child and indeed may be pleasurable. At least some patients view these experiences as neutral or positive. It is useful for the physician to focus primarily on determining which events occurred and how the patient reacted to them. The clinician is always aware that sexual abuse can produce serious psychopathology; nonetheless, one should not rush to judgment about its etiological significance.

WHAT INFORMATION DOES THE PHYSICIAN SEEK ABOUT ADOLESCENCE?

The period of development covered in this section is difficult to define in chronological terms. If adolescence is viewed as beginning when secondary sexual characteristics develop and extending to the time the individual assumes an adult role in society, this epoch can cover a range from the preteen years to well into the twenties. Ordinarily the clinician views adolescence as spanning the teenage years (from twelve to twenty). In taking this aspect of the patient's history, the clinician reviews categories of issues similar to those involved in the history of earlier childhood; one inquiries into the patient's family situation, schooling, extracurricular activities, and interpersonal relationships.

The major aspects of physical sexual development first became prominent in adolescence. This is an appropriate place for the clinician to inquire about the onset of menstruation and the patient's and parents' responses to this event. Questions can be asked about when secondary sexual characteristics began to appear, and how the patient and family members responded to these bodily changes. The physician is particularly interested in experiences of shame, being teased, or feeling different or "freakish" if rates of development varied significantly from the mean.

For most people, dating and sexual experience begin in adolescence. Questions should be asked about early dating experiences; in particular, were these encounters characterized by relative ease and comfort or by disabling tension and self-consciousness? If the patient is comfortable in discussing sexual material, the physician can also inquire into the extent of sexual activity during adolescence and whether sexual experiences were satisfying, coerced, frightening, or unpleasant. Patterns of homosexual preference may begin to emerge during this developmental period, and where relevant, the physician can inquire about homosexual fantasy and experience. Even if no homosexual experience took place, it is useful to know if the adolescent worried or had doubts about his or her sexual identity.

Most adolescents also have some experience with full- or part-time employment. The clinician can inquire about what kind of jobs patients had, how enjoyable or unpleasant they were, and how others judged their work performance. This is a time in life when patients may begin to think more seriously about the kinds of careers they will seek. These early work experiences may play a critical role in shaping their choices.

In American society, adolescence is a time when many individuals have their first experiences with mind-altering drugs. Inquiries can be made about the patient's first experience with alcoholic beverages and about subsequent patterns of drinking during adolescence. The patient should also be asked about use of cocaine, psychedelics, narcotics, sedatives, and amphetamines. Ordinarily, these inquiries can be made quite directly. Unless patients deny using any sort of drug, it is useful to run through a brief list of street drugs and ask specifically about their experiences with each. Most people are far more comfortable discussing their adolescent drug experiences than in revealing their adult patterns of drug use. Talking about drug abuse in adolescence may make it easier for them to acknowledge the presence of substance abuse problems in adulthood.

Adolescence is also a time when children appear to have more conflicts with their parents. The same child who is obedient, loving, and conforming during latency may in adolescence become argumentative, sullen, obstinate, and rebellious. Certainly, many adolescents adopt social views regarding religion, sexual, economic, and political issues that may be at variance with those of their parents. Some become worshipful of adults other than their parents, and the parents may view these idealized figures as less than satisfactory role models.

Much of adolescents' struggle with their parents may be an inevitable consequence of their need to develop a more independent existence, their new-found cognitive ability to be aware of the shortcomings of their parents, or their exposure to a different value system that is largely influenced by their peers. Whatever the causes, conflicts with parents during adolescence may engender painful feelings in both parties that are not easily resolved. The physician should inquire about events such as violent arguments, efforts on the teenager's part to leave the home, or long periods of drastically diminished communication between the adolescent and the parents.

Finally, the conflicts that adolescents have with their parents and society, their strong need for self-esteem, and their remarkable susceptibility to peer pressure increase their susceptibility to engaging in antisocial conduct. At this age, they are physically and psychologically mature enough so that society views such conduct as criminal and may take punitive action against them. It is useful to ask all patients if they were involved in minor delinquencies during adolescence, such as destruction of property, running away, or petty theft. If the answers to these questions are positive, further inquiries can be made into the possible history of more serious criminal activities, such as gang fighting or major theft. Although it is probably incorrect to view promiscuity as antisocial conduct, girls who are sexually active with multiple partners during adolescence are often so labeled. Usually, such sexual activities reflect a great deal of the adolescent girl's insecurity and her feeling that she can gain acceptance and recognition only through sex. If, as often happens, she is exploited in these activities, this exploitation will have a negative influence on her adult personality development.

WHAT ARE THE MAJOR ISSUES
EXPLORED IN THE ADULT HISTORY?

It is generally assumed that the learning experiences that individuals encounter after adolescence have a less powerful influence on shaping their adjustment than those encountered in earlier phases of development. Whether this is true or not, individuals do continue to have experiences that influence their mental health as they enter college or the work force, prepare for careers and marriage, raise children, and eventually enter middle and old age. The chronic sources of stress after adolescence are most likely to be related to problems with one's social role and with loved ones. Acute and traumatic stresses, such as severe accidents, the death of a loved one, or being the victim of an assault, may also elicit serious disturbances.

The main focus of the adult history is on the patient's occupational (including leisure), social (including sexual, marital, and child-rearing), and religious experiences. These are considered from the immediate postadolescent period up to the present.

The manner in which the patient's personality traits have developed and the impact that these traits have had and continue to have on the patient's environment are especially important. As patients discuss the manner in which they relate to work, leisure time, and loved ones, personality traits such as aggressivity, passivity, withdrawal, or dependency begin to be revealed. As a result, it becomes possible to understand how stresses in their lives emanate not only from accidental events and developmental expectations but also from how they deal with their environment. People burdened with maladaptive personality traits inevitably introduce a measure of stress into their lives. The paranoid person not only anticipates but, through his or her anger and suspiciousness, also helps to evoke a certain amount of animosity from the environment. Antisocial people are likely to create conditions that cause others both to distrust them and to respond to them sometimes in a punitive manner.

As the history of adult experience is reviewed, it is usually possible to determine which events and which personality traits have played a role in causing the patient's illness or complicating it. This aspect of the past history supplements material obtained in the history of the present illness and provides the examiner with a second chance to check out the details of how the illness developed. It should also be apparent that the history of adult experience merges into a consideration of the patient's current status. Indeed, as the adult history is reviewed, the details of the patient's symptomatology may be more carefully elaborated.

At this point in history taking, it is also useful to focus on the patient's positive attributes. One important reason for noting patients' past levels of accomplishment in work, creativity, or interpersonal relationships is that they provide a comparison with the current level of functioning. This comparison often gives some clue to the depth of their current illness and provides guidelines for anticipating how much improvement they are likely to make. Another reason for eliciting this information is that it helps suggest interventions that may increase the patient's self-esteem and sense of well-being. A depressed patient who has always been successful at manual tasks may find various aspects of occupational therapy useful during the process of rehabilitation. An elderly patient who has always relied on interpersonal relationships rather than private pursuits to obtain gratification will deal better with problems of depression or organic deterioration if he or she is provided access to environments in which there is significant contact with other people.

It is also true that some of the more severe mental illnesses begin after adolescence. In taking the adult history, the physician has a second chance to inquire into any history of previous illness. Some patients may not have provided this information when they were asked about it in earlier phases of the interview. A clinician dealing with a middle-aged person with a bipolar illness may find that the patient initially has little recollection of manic behavior during early adulthood. As the history of adult development is elicited in detail, however, recollections of earlier symptoms may return to the patient, or the physician may discover that there are lapses in the patient's past life that cannot be accounted for. Such lapses should lead the clinician to investigate whether the patient was seriously ill or perhaps even hospitalized during that time.

WHAT ARE THE MAJOR ISSUES TO BE COVERED
IN TAKING THE OCCUPATIONAL HISTORY?

If there is time, it is useful to go through the patient's entire work history from first job to the present. When time is limited, it may be more practical to ask what jobs the patient has worked at for the longest period of time and to focus more on the patient's present occupation. In either case, the physician should try to determine whether the status of patients' jobs, their degree of success at work, and the amount of energy they put into their work are static, increasing, or decreasing. Either upward or downward, occupational mobility can be stressful. The person who is doing well faces new obligations and challenges. The patient who is moving toward lower status occupations or who is doing a job less well must learn to deal with the realities of diminished power. Even if the patient's actual job performance remains static, it may be useful to inquire if it is getting more physically or intellectually taxing, or if it requires a greater expenditure of energy.

It is useful to spend a few minutes reviewing the exact skills that are required in the patient's current employment. This review helps the physician learn about various aspects of the patient's motor, social, and cognitive skills. (A receptionist needs to have a certain degree of social skill; a teacher can be expected to have an above-average level of intelligence and language skills.) Focusing on the details of the patient's job will also give patients a chance to talk about any work performance difficulties they may be having. Where patients have jobs that call for a high level of motor or cognitive capacity, the first effects of an organic brain disorder may be experienced at work.

If the patient's level of job satisfaction is high, it will help him or her to deal with a mental illness. If low, it may be a causative or complicating factor. Job satisfaction is determined by monetary rewards, the enjoyment of the work itself, and the quality of the interpersonal experiences available on the job. The physician should ask about each of these variables and will usually find that only one is necessary for job satisfaction. Corporate administrators may find their work stressful or boring but may be sufficiently gratified by their high salary to be satisfied. Musicians may work alone most of the time for very little pay, but their satisfaction is in the performance of the job itself. Bartenders may receive little compensation for relatively menial work but may thrive on their relationships with customers.

If patients report that their work is satisfying (and most patients do), it is useful to inquire if they view it primarily as a means to earn a living or as an end in itself. Some people view work as inherently rewarding, a career rather than a job. It provides them with a sense of meaning and identity. Not only is this true of those who do intellectual or creative work, but it is often equally true of those in service industries or those who elect to be homemakers. As they move toward middle or old age, patients' degree of commitment to their work may be an especially important factor in determining their stability. A woman who has devoted much of her energy to child rearing must make major changes in her self-image and daily activities when her children leave home. All people who view work as a career must make major adjustments when they retire.

Still other stresses associated with the work environment may be deleterious to the patient's health. Some factory jobs pose safety risks for the patient. Others may be carried out in highly noisy surroundings or may be so monotonous as to be oppressive. Sometimes, the work situation exposes the patient to chemical agents that impair brain function and produce symptoms of mental disorder. Patients who work in industries that manufacture insecticides, fungicides, batteries, glass products, or solvents are at risk of being exposed to neurotoxins such as lead, arsenic, carbon disulfide, and manganese. These substances can be etiological agents in a wide variety of psychiatric disorders.

Finally, it should be noted that the patient's current work situation may be a source of strength as well as stress. Even severely disturbed patients may be able to function quite well at work; indeed, they may find that work is the only satisfying aspect of their lives. The existence of a positive work situation may be a critical factor in the clinician's decision about whether or not to hospitalize the patient. Those patients who continue to enjoy work usually have sufficient psychological strength to be treated as outpatients. Here, the stress created by taking patients away from their jobs and putting them in a hospital may outweigh any advantages to be gained by inpatient treatment.

WHAT INQUIRIES SHOULD BE MADE ABOUT THE PATIENT'S EDUCATIONAL ACHIEVEMENTS AS AN ADULT?

Because many people in our society continue education after adolescence, it is useful for the clinician to inquire about adult educational activities. An awareness of educational achievement gives the physician clues to the patient's intelligence. It can be reasonably assumed, for example, that the patient who has graduated from college has relatively good intellectual abilities. Negative accounts are less informative; thus, it is not clear what a history of having failed to complete high school tells us about the patient's intelligence. Older patients from a rural setting may have quit school early to help support the family, and their lack of schooling may not at all reflect their intellectual abilities. Even positive accounts can be misleading. For example, younger patients from either rural or urban settings may have obtained a high school diploma on the basis of "social passing." Hence, although they have completed high school, they may have serious intellectual limitations.

Knowledge of the patient's past intellectual achievements allows the physician to compare them with the patient's current level of intellectual functioning. For example, a college graduate who has difficulties dealing with simple abstractions is likely to have a severe impairment. In a patient with limited intellectual capacity and limited education, a similar finding may have less clinical significance.

WHAT INQUIRIES SHOULD BE MADE ABOUT THE PATIENT'S MILITARY HISTORY?

A large percentage of males (and an increasing number of females) in our society have spent many months or years of their adult lives in military service. This is a unique environment for most people; in some ways, it is likely to be more stressful and, in some ways, less stressful than civilian life. Military service usually requires adjustment to a new geographical region while separated from family and friends. It also requires the capacity to live with very little privacy and in close proximity to members of the same sex, as well as an ability to adjust to a hierarchical culture in which one must submit to authority. Those who can make these adjustments are well taken care of. Their basic needs are met, and they are relieved of much of the stress involved in making choices about how they will spend their time. Some people find the adjustment to military discipline very difficult, and others are troubled by the loss of autonomy that military service imposes. Still others have difficulty with the change in their living circumstances and with their separation from loved ones. On the other hand, some people who have difficulty structuring their own lives as civilians may thrive in the military setting.

The military history reveals something about the patient's personality traits. It is always useful to inquire about how successfully the patient accommodated to military life and to obtain information about various military experiences. The rapidity with which patients advanced in rank provides a good index of the quality of their military adjustment. Inquiries into disciplinary infractions provide information about antisociality. Special attention should be paid to combat experiences and their subsequent impact on the patient. Veterans of combat and particularly those unfortunate enough to have become prisoners of war are susceptible to posttraumatic stress disorder. The physician will also want to inquire about any mental or physical problems that patients developed while in the service, and whether they have been adjudicated as having a service-connected disability. The latter fact may provide the patient with easy access to veterans' hospitals or with monetary rewards for disability.

WHAT INQUIRIES SHOULD THE PHYSICIAN MAKE ABOUT THE PATIENT'S LEISURE ACTIVITY?

Leisure time is valued and spent in a variety of ways. The career-oriented patient may have little interest in leisure pursuits, but other patients may view work only as a means of facilitating their spare-time interests. Leisure may involve activities such as sports, shopping, watching television, reading, listening to music, partying, working on crafts, home maintenance, building, or just spending time with friends and loved ones. A great many people prefer to spend their leisure time in the company of others, whereas others prefer to pursue leisure activities alone. Knowledge of how the patient spends leisure time may help the physician predict how the patient will respond to changes that may either compromise or expand leisure activity. It may also provide clues to planning rehabilitative interventions.

It is especially important that the clinician determine something about the quality of the patient's current free or leisure time. Is free time a period for relaxation, refurbishment, or joy, or is it a time of anxiety, boredom, or despair? One way to get at this information is to make inquiries about how patients spend their evenings and weekends. This line of questioning often allows them to talk about feelings of loneliness or depression. It is also a useful way for the physician to learn about current patterns of drug abuse. If asked how they spend a typical evening, patients who may deny excessive alcohol intake if asked about it directly may acknowledge that they have two or three cocktails before dinner and several bottles of beer afterward.

WHAT ISSUES DOES THE PHYSICIAN CONSIDER IN TAKING A SEXUAL HISTORY?

Most textbooks ritualistically stress the importance of the patient's sexual history. The approach here is that, unless patients complain of sexual dysfunction or are involved in a type of sexual behavior that troubles them or others, in the early phases of evaluation it need not be explored in great depth.

For the patient who reports no sexual difficulties, the effort to take a history of past sexual experiences may not provide sufficient diagnostic or therapeutic information to justify the invasion of privacy and the possible loss of rapport that it may produce. It is always possible, of course, that the patient is glossing over past difficulties, and that these will be revealed if the past sexual history is rigorously pursued. If there is sufficient time available, there may be justification for gently checking out the patient's assertions that there have been no problems. This should be done, however, only after a certain amount of rapport has been established.

There has been a significant change in attitude about sex since the 1960s, and many younger patients may be quite comfortable discussing sexual activities. Nonetheless, the physician should still be aware of the dangers of embarrassing the patient in the course of taking a sexual history. Questions should be asked matter-of-factly, and the patient's responses should be handled in the same way. Patients who seem reluctant to answer a question should not be pressed to reply. The preservation of a comfortable physician–patient relationship outweighs the value of whatever information is obtained under duress.

If the patient complains of long-standing sexual dysfunction, a more elaborate past history is required. In such cases, patients usually appreciate the need for a detailed inquiry into their sexual lives and are likely to be cooperative. Here, the clinician begins by determining if the major problem is lack of interest in sexual activity with available partners, or if the patient is aware of sexual desire but is unable to perform sexual intercourse satisfactorily. Chronic lack of interest may reflect abnormal physical conditions, chronic personality problems, or a learned fear of sexuality. It may also develop gradually as a response to performance problems. In evaluating diminished sexual interest, the clinician should inquire about sexual feelings that may be manifested in fantasy or dreams. Some patients engage in active masturbation with accompanying fantasies but cannot seem to become sexually involved with available partners. The clinician must also ask about nonsexual aspects of the patient's relationships with partners. Marital partners may lose sexual interest in one another when there are other problems within the marriage, particularly problems related to power struggles and feelings of not being valued by one's spouse.

It is especially important to investigate markedly diminished or absent sexual activity in older patients. Although most middle-aged and elderly patients continue to have gratifying sex lives, many do not. Not uncommonly, couples who marriages have been characterized by conflict markedly diminish or cease their sexual activities following the illness of one of the partners, the wife's menopause, or some crisis in the marriage. Although this cessation may be a major source of stress or grievance to one or both partners, eventually they adjust to the situation, give up on sexual activity, or seek it through another partner or masturbation. They may claim that they are not interested in sex and can do without it. Here, alleged lack of sexual interest may simply reflect a serious problem of communication within the marriage, where both partners have (incorrectly) accepted their lack of sexual activity as a sign of aging and have settled for what is often a quiescent but unfulfilling relationship.

If the patient expresses interest in sex with available partners but has had problems in performance, he or she should be routinely evaluated for a sexual dysfunction disorder. In addition to taking a history of recent physical illness and patterns of drug use, the clinician should inquire about when performance became a problem, what kinds of thoughts and feelings have compromised sexual enjoyment, and under what conditions sexual experience has been enjoyable. This information, together with information about other aspects of patients' relationship with their partner, forms the basis for treatment of their dysfunction. It may also alert the clinician to the possibility of an organic cause of the disorder.

It is good to keep in mind that many mental as well as physical disorders may be associated with sexual dysfunction. If patients present with symptoms of depression and inability to perform social or occupational functions as they have in the past, it is quite appropriate to ask them if they are also having some type of sexual dysfunction. Very often, they will reply affirmatively. Men will describe lack of interest in sex or lack of ability to perform the sexual act. Women will describe lack of interest, painful intercourse, or inability to reach orgasm. Once this information is obtained, it is useful to inquire about past sexual functioning. Conceivably these patients have had sexual difficulties that predate their present illness. If this is the case, more detailed exploration of past sexual dysfunction is appropriate. If the patient denies past difficulties, the clinician has learned that the patient's current difficulties represent a new symptom that is probably a manifestation of a mental or physical illness or a marital problem.

The issue of the patient's sexual preference may be obvious early in the interview. Some patients who are homosexual may acknowledge this fact in discussing their symptoms. No matter how comfortable patients may be with their homosexual orientation at present, it is safe to assume that it has caused them some painful moments in the past. Every homosexual must go through the process of realizing that his or her sexual preferences are different from those of his or her peers and is forced to deal with the many stresses that our society puts on those who prefer sexual partners of the same sex. The physician will want to ask about how the adjustment to homosexual preferences has influenced other aspects of the patient's life, and how it may be related to the current symptomatology. It is also useful to remember that homosexuals experience the same types of sexual dysfunction as heterosexuals and may need similar kinds of sexual therapy.

As inquiries about sexual activities are pursued or as other issues such as marriage and interpersonal relationships are discussed, the physician may come to suspect that a patient has homosexual preferences. If the clinician believes that it is important for the patient to talk about these preferences, the patient can be asked directly, "Have you ever had homosexual experiences?" or "Do you ever have homosexual fantasies?" It is useful to ask about past activities first because it is easier for the patient to acknowledge them. The patient who responds affirmatively can then be asked about current homosexual activities and preferences.

Still other patients, usually adolescents or young adults, may be very troubled by their homosexual orientation and may be struggling with various degrees of success to maintain heterosexual relationships. When this appears to be the case, the physician can again ask the patient quite directly about past and present experiences and fantasies. When patients are troubled about their homosexual proclivities, there is considerable controversy in psychiatry about the extent to which physicians should try to help them make a heterosexual adjustment. Certainly, in the evaluation phase, the physician should withhold judgment about what is the best outcome and should simply try to define the nature of the patient's sexual activities and motivations, as well as the extent to which they are a source of conflict. In this regard, the patient's masturbation fantasies often provide an important clue to what type of sexual orientation the patient will ultimately adopt.

In taking a sexual history, the physician also has the opportunity to learn about other important aspects of the patient's life. Sexual activities are intricately related to other interpersonal activities. Sex is likely to be used to gain power over one's partners or to gain attention or nurturance. The use of sex to gratify nonsexual interpersonal needs is usually evident to the physician. Men may talk about their need to have power over their partners. Women may discuss the use of sex as a means of controlling relationships. Women who have a poor image of themselves may be especially prone to use sex as a means of avoiding loneliness. Not uncommonly the so-called promiscuous woman does not enjoy the physical aspect of sex but feels she must be sexually active if she is to be loved by anyone. Such women are at high risk of being exploited by their sexual partners.

A final issue to be considered in taking the sexual history is the possibility that the patient has deviant sexual interests, such as voyeurism, exhibitionism, sadism, masochism, or pedophilia. Patients with these perversions or paraphilias may be sent for treatment because they are in trouble with the law, they may seek treatment because they fear legal difficulties, or they may be sincerely distressed by their deviant fantasies and aberrant behavior. It is also possible that a patient who seeks help for a nonsexual problem will discuss deviant fantasies or activities in the course of the interview. If the patient acknowledges deviant sexual motivations, the clinician's first task is to determine if these are gratified only through fantasy or by actual sexual conduct as well. Many people have highly deviant fantasies but do not act on them. If the patient has been acting on paraphiliac impulses in a manner that violates the law, the physician will want to seek detailed information about what kinds of situations elicit such actions, what aborts them, and the extent to which the patient can find gratification through socially acceptable behavior. These data are essential for instituting treatment programs that involve environmental control or behavioral therapy. It is also useful to obtain as much information as possible about the patient's early sexual experiences, as these may have etiological relevance.

WHAT ARE THE IMPORTANT ISSUES
TO BE EXPLORED IN THE MARITAL HISTORY?

These days, it is not uncommon for couples to live together for many years without getting married. Although these relationships have some qualities that are different from those found in marriage, for most purposes of psychiatric evaluation it is useful to view them as marriages. Another reality of modern life is that any patient over thirty has a high probability of having been divorced at least once. This means that the physician should be prepared to inquire about the history of marriages rather than "the marriage." The history of the marriage or marriages provides a picture of what are usually the most important relationships of patients' adult lives. Thus, it tells a great deal about patients' personality traits and their stresses, their vulnerabilities, and their patterns of learning during adulthood.

Once the physician has obtained data involving the courtship, the circumstances of the marriage, the length of the marriage, and the ages of children, questions can be asked about other aspects of the relationship. There are certain areas that are especially important, and these are listed and discussed briefly:

1. *The quality of communication within the marriage.* There is general agreement among psychiatrists that almost everyone's mental health is furthered by the opportunity to discuss feelings and problems with a loving, empathic person. Ideally, marital partners should be able to discuss freely with one another almost anything, particularly their feelings about one another. The beginning psychiatrist is often surprised to discover that many marriages are characterized by very limited communication. It is not only a matter of spouses keeping secrets from one another. Often, simple emotions such as anger, anxiety, or sadness are

never expressed or discussed. It may be even more surprising to the young psychiatrist to discover that marital partners do not always view their lack of communication as a problem and believe they have a good marriage. Although psychiatrists may make too much of the value of communication (and, conceivably, there are times when too much communication may be harmful), it is reasonable to assume that if a marital partner becomes mentally ill, the course and severity of the disorder will be influenced by patterns of communication with the spouse. Knowledge of how martial partners communicate may then provide guides for intervention through marital therapy.

The physician can learn about patterns of communication by asking the patient about them directly or by observing the patient in interaction with his or her spouse. As the patient reveals feelings such as anger or fear, it is appropriate to ask, "Have you shared this with your spouse?" If the patient answers negatively, the physician should inquire, "Why not?" The answer to this question is likely to clarify the limitations of communication that characterize the marriage.

2. *The frequency and quality of sexual relationships.* Taking the marital history provides the physician with another chance to learn about the patient's sexuality. The clinician will be especially interested in learning about any diminution or sudden increase in the frequency of sexual interaction. Changes in the frequency or quality of sexual activity may be associated with a mental or physical disorder, or with problems in the marriage such as conflicts or shifts in power within the relationship. Many men accept the idea of equality between the sexes intellectually but still find it difficult to deal with the reality of a wife's being assertive or, perhaps, being the main bread-winner. This may have a negative impact on their sexual interest and performance. Women who feel that they are being relegated to what they view as the low-status role of homemaker may similarly resent their husbands' successes in business, service, or academic careers. Such resentment may be expressed as a loss of interest in sexuality. Increased sexuality sometimes is a result of both partners' trying to salvage a marriage that is in danger of dissolution. Sometimes, a partner who is experiencing a manic episode seeks more frequent sexual activity and persuades his or her partner to comply.

3. *The quality of friendship between marital partners.* Some patients consider their spouses their "best friend." Both their nonsexual and sexual interactions may be characterized by a great deal of affection and playfulness. Such couples generally have many interests and activities in common. Other patients seem to view their spouses primarily as sex partners, bread-winners, or homemakers. The physician gets little indication of playfulness among these couples, who tend to focus on their marital obligations or duties rather than their marital pleasures. It is

almost always true that marriages characterized by playfulness and friendship are more stable than those that are not. Such marriages represent a more powerful source of support if one of the partners should become mentally ill.

The clinician can learn about this aspect of the marriage by asking such questions as "What do you and your spouse like to do together?" or "Do you play together very much?" or "Do you laugh at lot when you are with each other?"

4. *The capacity of the partners to retain separate identities.* In some marital relationships, friendship seems to be based less on playfulness or common interest than on a sense of desperation and need. The physician frequently sees patients whose marriages are characterized by an excessive degree of mutual dependency. Here, the couple may cling to one another for support, and each may be unconvinced of his or her capacity to be free of despair without the other being constantly present and available. Patients locked into this kind of marriage may be vulnerable to emotional distress should the other partner decide to pursue independent interests or become ill. The physician can learn about this marital pattern by asking questions such as "Do you have leisure interests that you pursue without your spouse?" or "How do you get along when you and your spouse are separated for several days?" Patients may respond to the latter question by statements such as "I am terribly lonely" or "I miss her very much." These comments may not be indicative of marital pathology. The type of comment that should engender more concern on the part of physicians is "We have never been apart for more than twenty-four hours," or "I just fall apart and go crazy when he's gone."

5. *The manner in which the spouse reinforces the patient's illness.* Some marital partners who otherwise show little affection may become quite attentive and compassionate when their partner becomes emotionally disturbed. If this pattern persists, patients may learn that they receive more gratification from their spouse when they are sick than when they are well. When symptoms are reinforced within the marriage, they become very resistant to most forms of treatment. Such symptoms may not be ameliorated until something is done to reeducate the spouse, usually in the process of marital treatment.

The physician can inquire about patterns of marital reinforcement directly by asking such questions as "How does your wife react when you have a headache?" or "Is she ordinarily that solicitous or attentive?" or "Do you enjoy her babying you even when you are not very sick?"

6. *The existence of patterns of exploitiveness within the marriage.* Although most marriages eventually reach some type of equilibrium in which the two partners' grievances and gratifications are approximately equal, there are some marriages in which one partner dominates and

takes advantage of the other. It is still common to see marriages in which women are ignored, treated like property, or brutalized by their husbands. Because of personality difficulties, religious beliefs, or lack of alternatives, these women may continue to endure the marriages. Such marriages may cause psychiatric symptoms or may worsen any pre-existing mental condition. The physician will usually pick up some hint that this kind of marriage exists when the patient is asked about the nature of the marital relationship and she describes her husband as domineering. At this point, it is useful to inquire if dominance is associated with physical violence. Sometimes, this question can be preceded by questions such as "Is your husband ever verbally abusive towards you?" or "Does he get more nasty when he's drinking?" Although physical abuse of women is the commonest type of brutality in marriage, the physician should not be surprised to find that, occasionally, male patients are physically abused by their spouses.

7. *The patterns of arguments within the marriage.* Some patients insist that they never argue with their spouses, and this assertion may be true. Sometimes, such a statement merely means that, when they discuss conflicts with one another, the couple try to mute their anger. When married people never argue, it is usually true that at least one partner is harboring strong resentment toward the other and would prefer a more open relationship. That person may be more susceptible to psychiatric symptomatology.

Arguments, of course, can also induce acute episodes of anxiety or sadness in one of the participants and can exert a corrosive effect on the marriage. Sometimes, such differences culminate in violence. For all of these reasons, the clinician is well advised to inquire about the content and form of marital disagreements. The content usually revolves around any combination of three issues: sex, money, and in-laws. (This statement, of course, is only a useful generalization. Some couples are quite creative in arguing about trivial issues related to power in the marriage.) Consistent patterns in arguing may be revealed by inquiries about what starts arguments, how long they last, what terminates them, whether they result in violence or reconciliation, and how they affect the participants afterward.

The relationships of patients with their children may also constitute a very significant source of stress or gratification in their lives. Raising a sick child or a psychologically difficult child puts great stress on a marriage and increases the risk of divorce. When children turn out to have physical or psychological handicaps, patients who have had strong hopes for their offspring may become bitter and may manifest sadness and depressive symptomatology. On the other hand, children provide hope for the future, a sense of immortality, and, for some patients, a "reason to stay alive."

The clinician should inquire about the ages and sexes of all children, any difficulties they may have had or are currently having, and the nature of their relationship with their parents. Many patients like to talk about their children and usually volunteer information readily in response to direct questions.

Although there are many patterns of family interaction that are believed to favor the development of psychiatric symptomatology, a full description of them is beyond the scope of this text. There is one pattern, however, that is so common and generally harmful that it deserves at least brief mention. This involves putting the child in a situation in which he or she provides gratification to one marital partner that more appropriately should be provided by the spouse. Such gratification is not usually sexual. Rather, children are more often asked to satisfy desires for intimacy and playfulness that are lacking in the marital relationship. Children placed in such roles may develop unrealistic views of their own power or excessive guilt. They may also be resented by the parent whose role they have partially usurped. One or both parents involved in this triangle may also experience symptoms, and there is a high likelihood of marital discord. It is always useful for the clinician to be alert to the existence of this pattern, which is likely to be uncovered as patients reveal their childhood history or describe the rearing of their own children.

WHAT INFORMATION SHOULD THE EVALUATOR OBTAIN ABOUT THE PATIENT'S RELIGION?

Religious beliefs add meaning to life and enable patients to deal with daily stress, tragedy, and the existential issue of death. They also play a powerful role in the development of one's conscience and value system. If patients belong to an organized church, religion can provide them with a community of involved people who may provide nurturance, or, conversely, may be a source of new stress. For all of these reasons, the religious history, which is often ignored, is a critical part of any psychiatric work-up. It is useful to inquire about the effect of religion on the patient's upbringing and about the kinds of religious beliefs and experiences patients have had throughout their lives. The clinician's knowledge of patients' current religious activities may be important in planning treatment. Many patients who have experienced past comfort and sustenance in religious activities may give them up when they become mentally ill. The clinician is usually wise to urge patients to resume these activities as soon as possible. Knowledge of the patient's religious belief may also influence treatment planning. Patients who have strong fundamentalist beliefs may not respond well to psychotherapies that emphasize expression of feelings, particularly anger, or that encourage confrontations.

It has always been difficult for me to understand why psychiatric clinicians are hesitant to take a religious history or to discuss spiritual issues with patients. Admittedly, there are patients who view some aspects of psychiatry, especially its psychoanalytic perspectives, as promulgating values that are inconsistent with their own. There are few such patients, however, and they can be treated with nonpsychoanalytic interventions. Even a psychodynamic approach may be successful with this group of patients. As they come to know the psychoanalytically oriented physician better, they may learn that there is not as much difference between religious and psychiatric values as they feared.

The key issue in taking a religious history is the physician's capacity to show respect for the patient's belief system. Although I belong to no formal religious organization, I do have a sincere interest in the way in which all persons seek to deal with the need to find meaning in their lives. Because of this interest, I have never had difficulty in pursuing religious inquiries with nonpsychiatric patients, even those who hold strict fundamentalist views.

All patients should be asked directly about the nature and depth of their religious beliefs. Those patients who deny religious beliefs can be asked, "Are there other beliefs that provide meaning for you or help you cope with issues such as tragedy or death?" Most people have thought about these issues and are willing to discuss them.

Beginning clinicians fear that a discussion of religion will lead to patients' asking them about their own religious beliefs. This fear is unfounded for two reasons. First, clinicians can simply elect not to talk about their own religious beliefs and can politely explain why they will not do so. Second, in many instances, there is nothing wrong with clinicians' revealing their religious beliefs. Even the question "Do you believe in God, Doctor?" can be answered directly. An affirmative response usually poses no problem for the patient. A negative response may initiate an interesting dialogue, particularly if the clinician is willing to acknowledge the importance of the search for meaning and his or her awareness that not everything about our universe can be scientifically explained.

FOR FURTHER READING

Anthony, E., and Benedek, T. (Eds.) *Parenthood: Its psychology and psychopathology.* Little, Brown, Boston, 1970.

Blos, P. *On adolescence.* Free Press, New York, 1962.

Bowlby, J. *Attachment and loss. Vol. 1: Attachment.* Basic Books, New York, 1969.

Boydstin, J. A., and Perry C. J. G. Military psychiatry. In *Comprehensive textbook for psychia-*

try (3rd ed.), H. I. Kaplan, A. M. Friedman and B. J. Sadock (Eds.). Lippincott, Baltimore, 1980.

Colarusso, C. A., and Nemiroff, R. A. *The race against time.* Plenum Press, New York, 1985.

Erickson, E. *Childhood and society.* Norton, New York, 1950.

Erickson, E. H., and Smelser, N. J. (Eds.). *Themes of work and love in adulthood.* Harvard University Press, Cambridge, 1980.

Gould, R. L. Adulthood. In *Comprehensive textbook of psychiatry,* Vol. 5. H. I. Kaplan and B. J. Sadock (Eds.). Williams & Wilkins, Baltimore, 1989.

Green, A. H. Dimensions of psychological trauma in abused children. *Journal of American Academy of Child Psychiatry,* 22:231, 1983.

Greenspan, S. J. Normal child development. In *Comprehensive textbook of psychiatry,* Vol. 5, H. I. Kaplan and B. J. Sadock (Eds.). Williams & Wilkins, Baltimore, 1989.

Lansky, M. R. (Ed.). *Family therapy in major psychopathology.* Grune & Stratton, New York, 1981.

Lewis, M. Psychiatric examination of the infant, child and adolescent. In *Comprehensive textbook of psychiatry,* Vol. 5, H. I. Kaplan and B. J. Sadock (Eds.). Williams & Wilkins, Baltimore, 1989.

Lidz, T. *The person.* Basic Books, New York, 1968.

Looney, J. G., and Oldham, D. C. Normal adolescent development. In *Comprehensive textbook of psychiatry,* Vol. 5, H. I. Kaplan and B. J. Sadock (Eds.), Williams & Wilkins, Baltimore, 1989.

McLean, A. *Work stress.* Addison-Wesley, Reading, Mass., 1979.

Minuchin, S. *Families and family therapy.* Harvard University Press, Cambridge, 1974.

Napier, A., and Whitaker, C. A. *The family crucible.* Harper & Row, New York, 1978.

Offer, D. *The psychological world of the teenager.* Basic Books, New York, 1969.

Ostow, M. Religion and psychiatry. In *Comprehensive textbook of psychiatry* (3rd ed.), H. I. Kaplan, A. M. Friedman, and B. J. Sadock (Eds.). Lippincott, Baltimore, 1980.

Roth, L. H. (ed.). *Clinical treatment of the violent person.* Guilford, New York, 1986.

Sadock, V. A. Normal human sexuality and sexual dysfunction. In *Comprehensive textbook of psychiatry,* Vol. 5, H. I. Kaplan and B. J. Sadock (Eds.). Williams & Wilkins, Baltimore, 1989.

Vaillant, J. E. *Adaptation to life.* Little, Brown, Boston, 1977.

CHAPTER FIVE

Evaluating the Patient's Current Situation and Personality Traits

In the course of taking the patient's recent history, the physician gradually moves into inquiries about the patient's current situation. The description of the patient's current situation could be viewed either as part of the history (the recent history) or as a separate and distinct aspect of the evaluation. The approach recommended here is that the clinician think about the various elements that make up the patient's present situation as a separate aspect of the evaluation.

As history taking draws to its conclusion, the clinician begins to consider how various personality traits may be expected to influence the patient's response to the illness and its treatment. There are a great many behavioral and experiential criteria that define personality traits. Some of these are also criteria for the personality disorder diagnoses listed in the DSM-III-R. Personality traits may also include dimensions of behavior or experience that are not usually viewed as symptoms of mental disorders. The patient's motivation, lifestyle, values, and views of himself or herself and the world can also be considered aspects of personality. In most neuropsychiatric textbooks, the development of information about personality is not considered a part of the mental status examination. The approach here is to view the evaluation of personality traits as a distinct aspect of the mental status examination. It is discussed separately only because such an evaluation requires a different approach to inquiry and observation than is required in the traditional neuropsychiatric mental status examination.

WHAT INFORMATION ABOUT THE PHYSICAL ASPECTS OF THE PATIENT'S CURRENT LIVING SITUATION SHOULD BE SOUGHT?

The physician should try to gain an overall picture of the patient's physical environment in terms of its location, the degree of comfort it provides, and how much access it offers to resources such as shopping, community centers, or churches. One critical issue that is frequently ignored by clinicians is how the patient's living arrangements may limit access to treatment. Some patients live a long distance from the clinic or hospital and have no easy means of getting there. In rural areas, this is a special problem for the poor or elderly who do not own an automobile or who cannot drive. In urban settings, clinical facilities are not always readily accessible by public transportation or may be located in areas where the elderly cannot safely travel.

Over one third of all appointments at mental health centers and public clinics throughout the nation are "no shows." There are many reasons, but a major one is that appointments are scheduled without adequate consideration of what resources the patient has for getting to them. Some patients try to please their doctor by agreeing to come at whatever time the doctor or clerical staff schedules their appointment, even when they know that they are unlikely to get there. Careful inquiry into patients' geographical situation and their resources for travel should encourage the clinician to schedule appointments more realistically.

It is obviously useful to know whether patients live in a trailer or a mansion, how much living space they have for themselves, what noise levels or levels of pollution they endure, what daily risk of violence they tolerate, and whether they have too much or too little privacy. Symptoms such as insomnia and anxiety are prominent in noisy environments. Isolation from people may exaggerate depression. In some neighborhoods where violence is endemic, seclusive behavior or reluctance to leave one's residence is caused by a realistic fear of assault and may not be a manifestation of a personality disorder or a phobic disorder.

Access to adequate shopping, recreational facilities, medical care, or the church of one's denomination may be severely restricted for the poor and the elderly. This restriction in itself may be stressful. It also limits the extent to which physicians can make recommendations for patients to become more involved with other people, to get more exercise, or to increase their level of structured activity.

WHAT INFORMATION SHOULD BE OBTAINED ABOUT THE PATIENT'S CURRENT INTERPERSONAL RELATIONSHIPS?

Most people relate regularly to a large number of other people. These relationships are with family members, friends, employers, other residents of institutions, co-workers, or those who deliver services, such as postal workers. The total group of individuals to which a person relates can be thought of as his or her social network. This network constitutes an environment that provides each person with certain levels of stimulation, care, and reinforcement. Learning about the patient's social network puts the physician in a better position to understand the stresses and supports generated by the current environment and how these may be modified in a helpful manner.

By the time the patient's recent history has been taken, the physician already knows a great deal about the patient's social network. Still, if the patient's current interpersonal situation is not considered separately, it is easy to miss valuable information. Patients may not volunteer information about the level of stress or gratification that their current social network brings them. One way to get at this information is to ask each patient about whom they interact with in a typical week, either directly or by letter or phone. It could take a long time for an active person with many acquaintances to answer this question. Here, the physician can sometimes save time by asking the patient to describe only those interactions that seem most important. With most patients, including those who are pleasantly surprised to discover how many people they interact with in a week's time, the extent and nature of the interpersonal network can be ascertained in a few minutes of interviewing.

In asking questions about the patient's interpersonal network, the physician should try to avoid embarrassing patients who may be ashamed of the paucity of their relationships. Such embarrassment may be particularly characteristic of the elderly, who often feel (correctly or incorrectly) that they have been abandoned by loved ones.

Some patients may wish to avoid talking or thinking about loneliness or may not want to acknowledge it as a cause of their discomfort. The physician can exert some influence on how openly the patient faces this issue. By responding to the patient's description of isolation with a matter-of-fact attitude and moving on to another subject, the physician can allow the patient to avoid discussing the most painful aspects of loneliness. On the other hand, if the physician is very empathic, patients may be willing to acknowledge the extent of their despair. The physician is best advised to gently follow the patient's lead. If the patient says, "Nobody ever calls but I don't mind, I have so much to do," it may not be wise to pursue the issue of loneliness. But if the patient says, "Sometimes the hours drag on, nobody ever calls, and nothing ever happens," inquiries such as "Do you worry if people care?" or "How do you try to deal with your feelings of loneliness?" or statements such as "That must be very painful" are appropriate.

WHAT QUESTIONS SHOULD THE PHYSICIAN ASK REGARDING THE PATIENT'S CURRENT ACTIVITIES?

The clinician is generally interested in the patient's current occupational stress and whether the extent of his or her current activity is gratifying. Workplace stress is related to changes in the nature of the job, to relationships with co-workers, or to the patient's possible loss of capacities. Patients who report that things are not going well at work should be asked specifically if there have been changes in their jobs. Often, these changes are determined by economic fluctuations. When certain industries do poorly, employees may fear for their jobs, or their work loads may be increased to an oppressive level. Inquiries should also be made about how patients are getting along with their supervisors, with those who work at the same level, and with those whom they supervise. Often, stresses are increased when a new figure enters the scene, someone who may be a supervisor who changes the rules or a peer whom the patient perceives as a rival. Stress created by deterioration in work performance can sometimes be detected by simply asking patients if routine tasks associated with their jobs appear to be getting more difficult. Where appropriate, evidence of the patient's diminished capacities can also be obtained from employers or co-workers.

If the patient has been unemployed for more than a few days as a result of illness or because of economic factors, the impact of this new status should be fully explored. Unemployment has many stressful consequences other than actual or feared loss of income. When family members whose social roles have been partially defined by their jobs cease going to work regularly, they may experience a profound loss of self-confidence and self-esteem. For many patients, too much inactivity is in itself a formidable stress. The rest of the family may also have a difficult time adjusting to the patient's lowered level of activity and constant presence in the home.

It is generally useful to ask the patient about all of his or her occupational and leisure activities during the past week. This inquiry may reveal that the patient is devoting an inordinate amount of time to work, is avoiding work responsibilities, or doesn't have enough to do. The clinician should pay special attention to reports of diminished leisure activity. Patients with mental disorders frequently cut back on leisure activities (such as visiting with friends or going to church) before they cut back on work activities.

WHAT ASPECTS OF THE PATIENT'S FINANCIAL AND LEGAL STATUS SHOULD BE EVALUATED?

One of the most troubling inequities in American society is our failure to provide all citizens with ready access to good medical care. This is an especially serious problem in psychiatry, where the choice, the locus, and the length of treatment may be largely determined by the patient's financial status. When patients are uninsured or have limited insurance, they have difficulty gaining access to treatments such as electroconvulsive therapy (ECT, which ironically was the "poor man's treatment" several decades ago), long-term psychotherapy, or medical detoxification. The above treatments may be unavailable at mental health centers or state hospitals, either because these agencies cannot afford to provide them or because they are subject to moralistic public pressure. (Antianxiety drugs are infrequently used in some mental health centers because of what is often an unrealistic concern about the risk of addiction. Nonmedical detoxification may be favored over gradual drug withdrawal in public institutions on the grounds that the patient who suffers the pains of withdrawal will learn a hard but beneficial lesson.)

Indigent patients can rarely choose a specific treatment; they must take what is offered or go untreated. There are also major inequities in the quality of hospital care. Private hospitals, ordinarily, far exceed public hospitals in terms of comfort and almost always have superior treatment facilities. Increasingly, the length of hospitalization is influenced by monetary considerations. Brief hospitalization is the rule for the indigent. As insurance companies increasingly restrict the number of hospital days they will pay for, only the wealthy can afford long-term hospitalization.

Aside from its obvious relevance to treatment, there are other reasons for wanting to know as much about the patient's financial status as possible. Lack of adequate financial resources is a major stress in American society. It may elicit symptomatology, and it is very likely to perpetuate it. On the other hand, money can provide gratifications that mitigate the pernicious impact of mental illness. Any clinician who has worked with both poor and wealthy patients soon learns that the wealthy usually do better. It may be that the same factors that result in a good prognosis also enhance the accumulation of wealth; a more parsimonious explanation is that money gives the patient access to better care and more control over the environment.

Most doctors are reluctant to ask patients about their finances, and many patients are unwilling to discuss them (in this decade, many patients seem more willing to discuss their sexual practices than their net worth). If the physician does not ask about finances, it is possible to make a rough estimate of the patient's income from knowing something about his or her job, education, and living arrangements or by observing his or her dress and mannerisms. Such cues, however, can be misleading. Patients who have high-paying jobs and many material possessions may be spending much more than they are earning and may have limited financial resources. On the other hand, the unemployed person or the laborer may have unsuspected access to financial resources. Most of the time, the clinician is well advised to ask patients directly about their finances and their ability to pay for treatment. Such questioning should not be a cause for embarrassment on the part of either the patient or the doctor. It is useful to remember that clerical staff (in either the private or the public sector) will ask the patient about money anyway. It is easier for the patient to respect a doctor who asks about money than to respect one who seems oblivious to it but makes sure that the secretary inquiries about it.

In considering how money affects patients' current experiences and control over their environment, questions such as "How much do you worry about money?" and "How has your financial situation affected your relationship with your spouse?" and "What would you change about your life if you had greater resources?" are appropriate. I have also found it useful to ask selected patients how they believe the sudden acquisition of a large amount of money (for example, a million dollars) would influence their symptomatology. Severely depressed or anxious patients usually insist that it would make no difference. Other patients may respond with interesting fantasies about how the lack of money may be influencing their symptoms, and these may provide clues to how external stress is indeed affecting their condition. Although this "million-dollar test" certainly does not distinguish various types of depression (it is not a psychosocial dexamethasone suppression test), it does offer the physician and the patient an easy entree to discussing the influence of money on symptomatology.

Another related financial issue is whether the patient is involved in litigation. With the astronomical rise in personal injury suits in our society, a very large number of psychiatric patients are involved in some kind of litigation process related to real or perceived injury. Often, the symptoms that patients bring to the doctor are elements of damages or harms that must be proved to exist before the patient is compensated. In the American legal system, the highest monetary rewards are provided to compensate for pain and suffering. As litigation drags on (it often lasts for five years or longer), those who are plaintiffs come to appreciate that higher financial awards are likely to be contingent on the degree of pain and suffering they continue to experience. If their legal adversaries insist that they are exaggerating their difficulties, they will be strongly inclined to prove that this is untrue. In such a situation, it is easy for patients to escalate symptomatology without even being aware that they are doing so. Litigation may then become a cause of, as well as a response to, psychiatric symptomatology.

Most patients are reluctant to discuss litigation with their doctors. The physician should, nevertheless, tactfully inquire about any diminution in the patient's quality of life or productivity following an accidental event or illness. Questions such as "It must have been a real economic hardship for you to have missed work for so long—how have you managed?" or "Did your insurance or the insurance of the person who harmed you cover all of your bills?" may provide openings for the patient to discuss litigation. The intent here is to help the patient talk about this issue without feeling that he or she is being accused of being greedy or of "faking" symptoms. If the physician believes that the fact pattern of the injury would have led to litigation in most situations, it may be useful to be even more direct and ask the patient if litigation has been considered. There is the possibility that this may plant ideas in the patient's head that were not there before, but the reality is that most patients have already thought about litigation.

WHAT ARE SOME GENERAL ISSUES THAT THE PHYSICIAN CONSIDERS IN EVALUATING PERSONALITY TRAITS?

The DSM-III-R defines personality traits as enduring patterns of perceiving, thinking about, and relating to oneself and to the environment. When we think about an individual's personality, we are concerned with the totality of these traits.

There are several reasons for evaluating personality traits. These traits may become so maladaptive that they constitute symptomatology in themselves. In the DSM-III-R, inflexible and maladaptive personality trait patterns are categorized as mental disorders. Even if personality traits are not so distressing or disabling as to be considered a manifestation of mental disorder, they will still exert a powerful influence on how the patient deals with symptoms and responds to treatment. These issues have already been discussed in Chapter One. The presence of maladaptive personality traits is also likely to increase the degree of stress in the patient's life. This is particularly true of traits that are expressed behaviorally, such as passive aggressivity, avoidance, impulsivity, or antisociality, where the behavior is likely to create adverse environmental responses. Finally, the physician can use knowledge of the patient's maladaptive personality traits to teach patients how to exert sufficient control over them so as to reduce the stressfulness of their lives.

The assessment of personality traits is based on history taking, on direct inquiries to patients about how they view their personalities, and on the physician's observation of how various traits are manifested in the psychiatric interview. The most difficult and, perhaps, the most important of these assessments is the observation of how patients interact with the physician during the interview.

The assessment of personality traits sometimes requires a great deal of inference on the part of the physician. This is particularly true of the clinician's observations of his or her interactions with the patient. One makes judgments about whether the patient's pattern of behavioral interaction rises to a level where it may be considered seductive, aggressive, or passive-aggressive; inevitably, such judgments are highly subjective. The clinician's decisions will be influenced by the standards or norms that he or she uses to define nondeviant behavior, and these, in turn, will be influenced by his or her past experiences. Efforts to discern persistent patterns of aberrant perception or thinking on the part of patients usually require even more inference, as patients may be unwilling or unable to describe their experiences. Even if atypical patterns of thinking or perceiving are revealed, the physician still must estimate the degree of their abnormality.

The assessment of personality traits is also complicated by the inconsistency with which the patient reveals them. A patient who appears to be aggressive and competitive in the first interview may turn out to be much more conciliatory and passive in subsequent interviews. Much of the presentation that the clinician observes will be determined by the patient's current level of anxiety, the nature of the interview, and the patient's perception of the evaluator. Furthermore, when the patient is suffering from a serious mental disorder, his or her personality traits are likely to be observed in exaggerated form. Not uncommonly, depressed or anxious patients show personality aberrations that disappear when their symptoms are alleviated.

For all of the above reasons, the clinician should be rather tentative in describing the patient's personality traits. Only traits that appear to be rather firmly established should be recorded. This is a good time for the clinician to use tentative phrases like "The patient appears to be seductive" or "At this time, the patient appears to be suspicious or argumentative" or "The patient describes himself as deeply concerned with accumulating wealth." Tentative comments avoid the mantle of certainty created by comments that aver that the patient *is* seductive, argumentative, or deeply concerned with accumulating wealth. Unless there is an obvious and primary personality disorder diagnosis, personality assessment should be viewed as an ongoing process that begins with speculations about the existence of various traits. Clinicians should be prepared to modify their views if greater familiarity with the patient proves that their initial impressions were wrong.

As noted earlier, psychiatric texts vary in their approach to personality assessment. Some emphasize the psychodynamic genesis of personality; others ignore the issue totally or simply assume that personality assessment is the job of the psychologist. The approach suggested here is that personality assessment is an important dimension of psychiatric evaluation, one that should be based on observations and inferences rather than offered as an explanation of the patient's psychopathology. In short, the approach should be phenomenological.

The clinician is urged to describe his or her observations and inferences as precisely as possible, without speculating about their etiologies.

The remainder of this chapter addresses the evaluation of those traits that are likely to increase significantly patients' *negative* interactions with the environment, or that are likely to have an important influence on how they respond to their disorders or to medical treatment. These traits will be divided into two categories, which may, at times, overlap; those that are primarily behavioral and that are assessed on the basis of the history and from observations made during the interview, and those that are primarily related to the patient's patterns of thinking, which are assessed on the basis of the patient's own self-reporting as well as from the history and from inferences made during the interview. Unless there are many interview hours available, it is unlikely that the physician will learn a great deal about all of the personality traits to be considered below. The physician's task is to try to define the most obvious and salient traits and to describe them briefly in the record.

Because there is ongoing controversy about the validity of the categories of personality disorder listed in the DSM-III-R, and because most patients have a variety (rather than a single set) of dysfunctional personality traits, I have elected simply to discuss important traits without regard to how they may define mental disorders. The reader who is familiar with the DSM-III-R will also note that some of the traits discussed here are different from those discussed in that manual.

WHAT ISSUES DOES THE PHYSICIAN CONSIDER IN EVALUATING THE BEHAVIORAL MANIFESTATION OF PERSONALITY TRAITS?

The Patient's Attractiveness

Although there is no scientific way to measure qualities like charm or likability, these traits do have a powerful influence on how people live their lives, on how comfortable and happy they become, and on how they respond to emotional disorders. The history will reveal something about the patient's attractiveness to others; this trait, however, is most easily observed in the physician–patient interaction. Some patients are a pleasure to be with from the first moment. Others are unpleasant or make the doctor uncomfortable. Physicians are usually attracted to patients who show evidence of warmth or caring for others, who have a wide range of interests and a fertile imagination, and who can retain a sense of humor even while suffering from a mental disorder.

The presence of the above traits generally help patients cope with their mental disorder. Attractive patients are likely to keep their support systems intact even when they are in great distress. Unfortunately, attractiveness can also be used to hide symptomatology or to manipulate the physician into behaving in nontherapeutic ways. Patients who do not want to reveal the extent of their suffering or disability to the doctor may cover up their difficulties by being excessively friendly or witty. They may distract the physician by demonstrating their knowledge about their illness or about other subjects that they sense are of interest to the doctor. Other patients use their charm to maximize the doctor's attention and concern. The physician must also be alert to patients who use their charms to try to seduce him or her into nontherapeutic acts such as prescribing unnecessary drugs, allowing premature passes or discharges from the hospital, or becoming sexually involved with them.

Controllingness

Power struggles are ubiquitous in human relationships, even among people who are fond of one another. Everyone wishes to exert a certain degree of control over how others interact with him or her. Most people, however, realize that they cannot fully control their interpersonal environment, and that they must share power with others. Patients who regularly try to exert control over others may use a variety of means for doing so. Some will threaten or actually cause physical harm. Others exert control through willfulness. They demand that things be done their way and stubbornly resist compromise. Others gain control by assuming leadership roles and by claiming the power that accrues to those who have the greatest responsibilities. Patients who have less obvious sources of power may still exert control in relationships by withdrawing, or threatening to withdraw, affection if they do not get their way, or by being manipulative or seductive. Still other patients, who are sometimes described as having passive-aggressive traits, gain a certain degree of control by merely failing to comply with the demands of others. (This trait will be discussed further in another section.)

Although judgments about controlling tendencies require a high level of inference, they are worth making. Any personality trait that is associated with an excessive quest for power is likely to diminish the quality of interpersonal relationships. In whatever form this trait is expressed, it is likely to be a factor in eliciting symptoms or in aggravating or sustaining them. The patient's excessive need to control the doctor–patient relationship may also compromise treatment.

Information about the patient's inclination to control is often obtained in the process of taking a marital or sexual history. It can also emerge from the patient's work history or from aspects of the family history. Questions such as: "How do you resolve arguments in your family?" or "How do you discipline your children?" or "How do you get along with your boss or those who work for you?" may help the patient reveal aspects of control orientation.

The physician can also learn about the patient's need to control by observing how the patient interacts with him or her in the interview. Some patients are demanding and forceful even when they are miserable. Others exert control in the interview by not answering certain questions or by answering them insufficiently or inaccurately. There are patients who try to gain control over the relationship by, in effect, interviewing the doctor and seeking to reverse roles. Still other patients may try to exert control by talking continuously or by being seductive. The arrogant patient will sneer at certain questions as obvious or "psychiatric" or irrelevant; only preferred topics will be permitted. The paranoid will control by questioning the doctor's motives — or character. The narcissist will control by deviousness, manipulation, boasting, and lying.

Dependency

Human beings are interdependent and must, at times, rely on others to take care of their emotional and physical needs. Too much dependency, however, compromises a person's wish for other gratifications, such as a sense of freedom, autonomy, or power. There is no firm line that defines when a person is too dependent on others; moreover, making this judgment is complicated by the fact that an individual's dependency needs change as the person moves through various stages of development. Nevertheless, patients whose lives are characterized by little power or autonomy and by obviously excessive reliance on the power of others are at high risk of suffering mental distress and disability. These patients view themselves as having little capacity to change their lives and appear helpless in the face of stress.

Dependent behavior is, of course, common in people who are sick. For this reason, the doctor cannot assume that patients who plead for help, who appear submissive, or who proclaim that they can do nothing to influence their illness have strong dependent personality traits. Some patients appear to be quite helpless and dependent in the acute phases of their illness; when their symptoms recede, however, they may quickly demonstrate more autonomous behavior. It is only when this trait was consistently present before the patient became symptomatic that patients can confidently be viewed as being excessively dependent.

As a general rule, dependent patients are difficult to treat. They quickly learn that their symptoms bring them a great deal of gratification of their wishes for dependency. Such gratification may becomes a powerful reinforcer of symptomatic behavior. Although dependent patients may insist that they wish to be symptom-free, they are often reluctant to abandon the sick role. At the same time, they are generally cooperative in taking medications and following the physician's suggestions. Because of the gratifications they experience in the sick role, however, they may not respond to treatment as rapidly as the physician would hope.

Passivity

People vary in the manner in which they cope with the demands of life. Those who tend to be "doers" take an active stance in confronting problems or stress. As long as a person is truly capable of influencing the environment, this is an adaptive quality. Others, particularly those who also have dependent traits, perceive themselves as having little control over events. They move through life as though they are always at the mercy of the environment. These individuals seem to endure rather than cope. Sometimes, they endure to the point of continuing to live with painful emotional responses to stress.

There are some situations in which passivity may be adaptive. Prisoners, for example, or any oppressed group usually make a more satisfactory adjustment if they accept their environment as unchangeable. For most adults living in a free society, however, passivity is maladaptive. Those who are too passive may fail to deal with situations that can actually be changed. Such people do not cope effectively with the external stresses related to their illness, nor are they likely to participate effectively in treatments (such as psychoanalytically oriented psychotherapy) that require them to assume a certain degree of initiative.

Although passive persons do not actively attempt to change their environment, they are not without influence on it. Those who simply fail to fulfill reasonable demands for adequate social and occupational performance create a certain amount of difficulty for others. Resistance to legitimate environmental requirements is called *passive-aggressive behavior* because it is usually designed to express covert aggression toward others. Passive-aggressive persons procrastinate, dawdle, and forget when demands are made on them, and they usually complain that the demands are excessive. Their relationships, particularly with those who have authority over them, are troubled. Not surprisingly, these patients may resist cooperation with the physician's plans for treatment.

The physician discovers evidence of passivity or passive-aggressiveness primarily by reviewing the history of the patient's interpersonal relationships. These traits are also likely to become manifest in the doctor–patient relationship but may not be immediately apparent. Often, the physician cannot observe the patient's passivity or passive-aggressiveness until the patient has demonstrated an unwillingness to take an active role in the treatment process or has resisted the physician's advice or suggestions.

Aggressiveness

The term *aggressiveness* has several meanings. Sometimes, it refers to violence or the use of physical force with the intent of causing harm. Frequently, the term is used to characterize verbal behavior that is demanding, insulting, or threatening, and that appears intended to cause others psychological distress. Sometimes, the term is used to characterize competitive or assertive behavior that, although self-serving and perhaps troubling to others, is not intended to harm.

Verbal or physical aggressiveness is usually associated with the emotional experience of anger. This link is so close that, most of the time, we automatically assume that the aggressive person is angry. Therefore, it is convenient and probably necessary to evaluate the patient's inner experiences of anger at approximately the same time as its behavioral manifestations are explored. There are two clinical realities that complicate this type of evaluation. First, anger is not always expressed behaviorally. This means that the clinician must be concerned about how the patient deals with the emotion of anger when it is not expressed. Second, some patients may be aggressive (usually verbally) without being aware that they feel angry. These patients may have difficulty controlling their aggressiveness, and its apparent inappropriateness may elicit highly negative responses from others.

In evaluating both the experiential and the behavioral aspects of anger, it is useful for the clinician to begin by determining if the patient recognizes when he or she is angry. Patients differ in the extent to which they experience anger. Many patients have been trained to avoid acknowledgment of angry feelings by parental and religious admonitions that teach that it is morally wrong to be angry. The patient's failure to recognize and experience angry feelings may produce or exaggerate other painful emotions, such as anxiety or depression. It may also place the patient at a disadvantage in dealing with interpersonal situations in which anger is appropriate. If the patient does acknowledge the. experience of anger, the physician's task is to inquire about how the patient responds to it. It is important to inquire whether the patient deals with the experience by having a temper tantrum, sulking, withdrawing, or informing the appropriate individuals directly about the fact that he or she is angry.

The physician tries to determine whether the patient experiences anger appropriately by noting instances in the patient's history in which he or she has been treated rudely, has been taken advantage of, or has been physically or verbally abused by others. The examiner can then ask questions such as "How did you feel about that?" or "What were your feelings when he insulted you?" If patients deny experiencing anger, it is sometimes useful to make it easier for them to acknowledge it by remarking, "Most people in your situation would have been very angry. Is there any reason why you were not?"

When asked about feelings engendered by others' treating them badly, patients of fundamentalist background often respond by stating, "I was hurt, not angry." There are many ways of viewing such a response, but perhaps the most useful is that the patient was aware of strong and unpleasant emotions but was unwilling to identify them as anger. This denial of anger may take on absurd proportions (e.g., "I wasn't angry when she had an affair with my best friend. I was just hurt"). When encountered, as a rule such a degree of denial cannot be effectively challenged during the evaluation phase of the doctor–patient encounter.

If the patient acknowledges the experience of anger, the physician's task is simply to ask, "How do you deal with that feeling?" The patient's response will provide clues to patterns of dealing with anger that may be maladaptive. Ordinarily, the adaptiveness of a given response to anger varies with environmental circumstances. There are times when expressing even righteous anger is unwise (e.g., when a police officer is rude to one or when an employer has incorrectly criticized one). Here, the best solution may be a "cool" response to the immediate situation followed by "letting off steam" to a friend, or going home and exercising, or getting absorbed in work or a hobby. On the other hand, there are many more common situations in which others will respond in an understanding or conciliatory manner if they are simply informed of the patient's anger. Here, a direct statement such as "I am upset and troubled by your actions" can be made without escalating conflict. As a general rule, shouting, threatening, sulking, withdrawing, or attempting to make others feel guilty are maladaptive responses. Many patients (and some clinicians) make the mistake of equating the expression of anger with highly dramatic behavior such as shouting, threatening, or violent action. Patients need to learn that this means of expressing anger is almost never adaptive, and that anger that is expressed calmly and conversationally is most likely to elicit a rational and corrective response from others.

Verbal aggressiveness expressed in an inappropriate context may be quite maladaptive. One such context is the psychiatric interview. There are a number of reasons why a patient may express verbal aggression toward the doctor. Psychotic patients may misinterpret the physician's role and motivations. Less disturbed patients may respond to anxiety generated in the interview situation by becoming demanding, confronting, or even insulting. If this response to anxiety is repetitive, it can be viewed as a manifestation of a personality trait. Ordinarily, the physician can simply observe such behavior or make some remark about it and ask the patient if it occurs in other contexts. However, if verbally aggressive behavior exceeds the physician's level of tolerance or appears to be compromising the usefulness of the interview, the physician must call it to the patient's attention and insist that the patient try to behave more appropriately.

It is important that the doctor distinguish between reasonable assertiveness and aggression. The patient who is very direct in asking about the physician's training, fees, and prescriptions, or who refuses to discuss certain issues may be acting adaptively, even if he or she does not show the level of reverence or respect that the physician has come to expect. Such assertiveness on the patient's part may turn out to be a manifestation of inappropriate aggressiveness, but it is a mistake to label it this way prematurely.

The physical expression of anger or violent behavior is highly maladaptive. The person who threatens violence or becomes violent is unlikely to sustain successful relationships; sooner or later, such a person will elicit punitive responses from the environment. Under extreme circumstances, almost anyone can become violent; however, some patients are especially apt to resort to violence in the face of minor stress. Repeated violent behavior is appropriately viewed as a personality trait. It is seen in patients who have failed to develop more effective ways of dealing with emotions such as anger, anxiety, or sadness.

There are often urgent reasons for the physician to evaluate the patient's violent tendencies. In some clinical situations, the physician may be concerned that the patient will be violent toward him or her. In a much broader variety of clinical situations, the physician must be concerned that the patient may, at some time in the near future, be violent toward another person. Here, the physician is called on to predict the likelihood that a patient will commit a violent act, and if that likelihood is high, the doctor is obligated to try to hospitalize that patient, even involuntarily.

The issue of predicting imminent violence (or suicidality) will be discussed in subsequent chapters. Here, only the assessment of violence as a personality trait (which is certainly one aspect of the predictive process) is considered. This assessment is based primarily on the patient's history. Where the patient describes fear of losing control, has threatened others, or has a history of impulsivity, inquiries about past violence should be routine. Patients can be asked directly, "Have you ever used physical force to get your way?" or "Have you ever accidentally or intentionally hurt anyone?" This type of questioning can be repeated as various phases of the patient's life are explored. It is also important to determine what type of internal experience and environmental events preceded and followed any violent act. Knowledge of antecedent and consequent events helps the clinician to predict or prevent future violence.

Sometimes, patients deny past violence, but the physician believes it has occurred. To explore this belief, the physician can gently investigate the possibility of past violence by asking patients if they ever experience angry feelings toward people who have hurt them or have taken advantage of them. This line of inquiry can be followed by a question about whether they have ever wanted to harm such persons physically. At this point, such patients may acknowledge past violence. There are, of course, many reasons why patients may wish to be dishonest in discussing violent behavior, and often, information about violence can be obtained only from more objective sources.

Competitiveness is assessed by noting instances in the history in which the patient has competed appropriately, has avoided competition, or has been relentlessly competitive. Patients who avoid competition may miss out on opportunities for material and interpersonal gratification. Patients who are overly competitive tend to alienate others. The physician obtains data about competitiveness both from the history and by asking patients directly how they have responded to competitive situations. Ordinarily, patients who are competitive at work are also competitive in leisure activities. Patients may also compete in their interactions with the physician; thus, they may seek to demonstrate superior verbal skills and knowledge. Although such competitiveness may be peculiar to the interview situation, it is usually wise to assume that such patients behave similarly in other contexts.

Attention Seeking

All people want to have their positive qualities and accomplishments noted by others, but there are some people who seem driven to seek social attention. This trait is more likely to be observed in the process of evaluating than to be described in the history. The physician often encounters patients who spend a great deal of time trying to impress him or her with their importance or worth. These patients sometimes appear to be more interested in impressing the physician than in receiving help. They may brag, exaggerate, and strive to be entertaining, or they may be frankly seductive. As a rule, patients who try to impress the physician are likely to exhibit the same behavior in other interpersonal relationships. Sometimes, this can be observed in their interactions with others or by interviewing relatives or friends. The patients themselves, however, may be unaware of this type of conduct.

Other patients appear to be seeking attention in less direct ways. They may bombard the physician with many complaints and demands for help. Often, they make demands for special care, such as meeting only at certain times or under certain circumstances. Even when their behavior is abrasive, it seems designed to call the physician's attention to their specialness. Patients who tend to seek the physician's attention through demandingness and symptomatology may not evidence similar patterns of conduct in other relationships. This form of attention seeking is sometimes an artifact of the clinical situation; the doctor is viewed as a special and powerful person whose continuous attention is essential to the patient's well-being. The patient may have shown similar patterns of conduct with other "special" people in the past as well as currently but is not likely to show this pattern with everyone.

The forms of attention seeking described above are commonly seen in patients with histrionic, narcissistic, antisocial, and borderline personality disorders. This trait is often associated with unreliable reporting and exaggeration of symptoms. When present, it makes the physician's task of accurately defining the nature and severity of the patient's illness more difficult. It also makes it more difficult to treat such patients or to assess their progress.

Exploitiveness

In taking the history, the physician generally obtains clues to whether the patient's relationships have been characterized by a certain degree of mutuality or if they have been typified by exploitiveness. Some patients regularly seem to use people to gratify their own needs while doing very little to gratify others. As they present their history, they may show little evidence of kind feelings or behavior toward family members or friends. When they try to impress the physician with their concern for others, their statements do not ring true. As they talk about unsuccessful relationships, they emphasize how others have failed to provide for their needs and they minimize uncaring or overcontrolling conduct on their own part.

Of course, patients do not with to present themselves as exploitive, and a great deal of inference is involved in postulating that they are. The presence of this trait is most comfortably ascertained if there is objective history of its presence, or if the patient attempts to treat the physician in an exploitive manner.

There are other patients who seem to create situations in which others take advantage of them. As they describe their many unsuccessful relationships, they convey a sense of having repeatedly become involved with exploitive individuals and of doing little to resist being taken advantage of. Some of these patients complain about their bad luck. Others take a paranoid stance and blame their plight on the malevolence of those who exploit them. Still others recognize that they allow themselves to be exploited but don't know what to do about it. This trait is usually apparent from history taking alone, and objective verification may not be necessary.

Patients who assume either exploitive or exploited roles in their interpersonal life do not develop satisfying and consistent relationships. When they encounter difficulty in life, they are unlikely to have reliable sources of support. This situation, in turn, may lead to their having an unusual degree of difficulty in coping with their symptoms and a less than satisfactory response to psychiatric treatment.

Patterns of Privacy

Although people seek intimacy, they do not wish to be intimate with everyone and sometimes do not wish to be intimate at all. At times, in fact, they want to be alone. For most people, privacy provides a respite from the stresses inherent in monitoring their interpersonal behavior. It allows them to move "offstage," so that they can contemplate, reflect, and plan future actions. People vary enormously in their perceived needs for privacy. Some individuals are most at ease and most content when alone. Others may be frightened of being alone; in any case, they structure their lives so that they are almost always surrounded by people. The adaptiveness of these traits varies with the environment. In an institutional setting, such as an army barracks, for example, the person who prefers privacy is at a distinct disadvantage. On the other hand, those who constantly seek the company of others may have difficulty accepting the increasing isolation that is often associated with aging.

Too much isolation or too much dependence on the stimulation of others handicaps the patient in dealing with the stresses of everyday life or of illness. Either trait may also create new stresses that may play a role in the etiology of a mental disorder. Understanding the manner in which the patient seeks or avoids privacy also provides clues to treatment. Patients who are too isolated will benefit by environmental change that increases interpersonal contact with others. Patients who are highly dependent on the stimulation of others may have to be taught ways of tolerating and enjoying aloneness.

The attitudes of patients toward aloneness or privacy are ascertained on the basis of their own statements and their past history. It is important here to distinguish between attitude and behavior. There is a difference between seeking privacy and having it thrust on one. Some patients who present a history of relative isolation may have actively sought and welcomed it. Other patients fear being alone and may suffer profound experiences of loneliness and sadness as a result of isolation.

WHAT ISSUES DOES THE PHYSICIAN CONSIDER IN EVALUATING ASPECTS OF PERSONALITY ASSOCIATED WITH PATTERNS OF THINKING?

How people think has a powerful influence on how they feel and behave. A major school of psychiatric treatment, cognitive therapy, is based on carefully elucidating the content of patients' thoughts, particularly thoughts about themselves or others; determining how incorrect patterns of thinking adversely affect their emotions and behavior; and then helping them to develop more adaptive ways of thinking. Psychiatric disorders characterized by symptoms of anxiety and depression are better understood and more effectively treated if the clinician is able to discover how patients think about themselves and other people, about material possessions, about secular and spiritual issues, and about their illness.

The Patterns of Thinking about Oneself

All individuals have an internal image of their physical, behavioral, and experiential attributes. This self-assessment (usually referred to as the person's *self-concept*) varies with environmental circumstances but also has a great deal of consistency. Self-assessments tend to have a judgmental quality. We like certain aspects of our body and not others. We approve of some of our motivations and fantasies, and we are ashamed of others. We approve of some of the ways in which we interact with people, and we disapprove of others.

The physician is especially concerned about negative self-appraisals. Many patients have repetitive negative thoughts about themselves, such as "I am too fat," "My body is ugly," "I am selfish," "I am incompetent," "I am lazy," or "I am basically unlovable." Negative thoughts can, of course, be a product of a depressed mood, but they often antedate clinical symptoms of depression and may actually increase the severity of unpleasant emotional states. They may also influence behavior and handicap the patient's efforts to develop gratifying relationships with others. In fact, negative self-assessments tend to be inaccurate. Many mentally ill persons are likely to assess themselves more negatively than a truly objective observer might. Correcting these erroneous self-appraisals may have a powerful therapeutic effect.

The physician begins the assessment of the patient's self-concept by noting any statement that patients make about themselves, such as "I'm really a very sensitive person," "I'm a very competitive person," or "I never feel as if I'm worth anyone's attention." Next, the physician tries to make some judgment about the accuracy of patients' views. One way to do this is to ask patients more questions about their statements, about themselves, such as, "In what ways are you selfish?" or "Do other people find you so aggressive?" or "Why do you believe you are ineffectual?" It is then helpful to consider how congruent patients' self-concepts are with other data about them. The past history and other observations made during the interview may contradict negative self-assessments. A person who has had a distinguished career and is brought to the hospital by obviously concerned relatives is likely to be inaccurate if he insists that he is worthless and nobody cares about him. It is useful to ask friends or relatives questions about their view of the patient. Not uncommonly, they have a different and more positive view of his or her attributes.

The physician can also estimate the extent to which the qualities that patients describe as characteristic of themselves are also observable in the interview. Patients who state that they are always gentle and passive, and who come across as angry and demanding, are likely to be perceiving themselves inaccurately. Patients who describe themselves in highly negative ways often come across as quite likable. It is reasonable to assume that their self-concepts are unduly negative and are playing some role in creating or sustaining their symptomatology.

Sophisticated patients who are not very disturbed can be asked more direct questions about their self-concept, such as "What kind of person are you?" or "How would you describe yourself?" or "What do you see as your strengths and weaknesses?" or "What do you like best about yourself?" or "What do you like least about yourself?" They can also be asked how they would like to be different, or what their ideal self-image is. As patients define the differences between their self-concept and their idealized sense of self (sometimes called the *ego ideal*), the clinician can make a rough estimate of their degree of discontent or unhappiness.

In addition to assessing themselves, patients also have ideas about how other assess them. If patients respond affirmatively to the question "Do others see you as you see yourself?" they are confirming the accuracy of their self-concepts or are distorting both their self-concepts and how others perceive them. Additional observations of past history and interview behavior will be necessary to make these distinctions. If, however, patients report that others see them differently than they see themselves, the clinician should ask, "What do you think accounts for these conflicting views of what you are like?" Some patients acknowledge that others may be more accurate observers, and that their own view of themselves is distorted. Other patients insist that their own views of themselves are accurate, and that others are simply being misled or deceived.

Patterns of Thinking about Others

In an earlier section, aspects of the patient's manner of relating to others, such as aggressiveness, passivity, controllingness, or dependency, were discussed as behavioral manifestations of personality traits. It is likely that certain consistent patterns of thinking are associated with each of these behavioral patterns. In the time allotted for most evaluations, however, the clinician may not learn a great deal about most patterns of thinking associated with behavioral traits and can only speculate about them. There are some aspects of the patient's thinking about other people, however, that can be roughly assessed in a brief evaluation. These are related to the accuracy with which patients assess the attributes of others and the degree to which patients understand how they influence and are influenced by others.

Patients commonly misperceive the intentions of others. This can be a formidable handicap that may have major behavioral consequences. Those who perceive and anticipate too much benevolence on the part of others often find themselves taken advantage of. Those who are too suspicious may end up alienating others. Attitudes of irrational trust may be associated with a history that includes examples of the patient's being taken advantage of. Sometimes, the physician is alerted to such a pattern by observing that the patient appears to have a degree of unconditional trust toward him or her that goes beyond realistic expectations. A few patients directly discuss their belief in the inherent goodness and reliability of others.

Patients who are overly suspicious of others generally express resentment of what they perceive as exploitation. They may verbalize concern that the malevolence or ineptness of others forces them to live their lives cautiously. Some very suspicious patients may be unwilling to talk about their suspicions directly but may evidence their attitudes in relationship to the physician. A certain amount of distrust of physicians, especially psychiatrists, is not unusual in our society. But when patients repeatedly ask questions such as "Why do you want to know that?" and "What are you going to do with this information?" demand to learn as much as they can about the physician's qualifications, or refuse to respond to innocuous questions, it is reasonable to assume that their suspicions are high and exceed the bounds of appropriate cautiousness.

Patients may also have difficulty in estimating the strengths, weaknesses, or attractiveness of others. One common pattern is for patients to idealize some individuals, to denigrate others, and to allow for little middle ground. Such patients often show inconsistent and unstable attitudes toward the same individual. A once-idealized person who fails to meet their expectations may quickly be relegated to the ranks of those who are viewed as malicious, insensitive, or weak. This pattern of polarizing estimates of others (sometimes called *splitting*) is an important feature of some of the more severe personality disorders; it is obviously not conducive to forming stable and gratifying interpersonal relationships.

Sometimes, patients are aware of their tendencies to over- or underestimate the strengths, weaknesses, or attractiveness of others or to change their assessments of others' strengths rapidly. More often, the physician uncovers maladaptive patterns of estimating others by listening for evidences of such behavior in past relationships. It may be useful to ask questions such as "Do you have a tendency to hero-worship or idealize others?" followed by the question "Do you generally sustain your early positive view of others, or do you tend to be quickly disappointed in them?"

Many patients idealize physicians and endow them with capacities that they do not possess. This attitude is usually apparent in the degree of reverence, warmth, and compliance the patient demonstrates during the interview. The physician can use patterns of idealization to some advantage in eliciting the patient's cooperation; however, the physician must be wary of the possibility that such idealization also heralds a prolonged dependent relationship or a rapid shift to an attitude of anger and betrayal if the treatment does not go well.

An important factor in dealing with the interpersonal environment is knowledge of how one comes across to and influences other people. Such knowledge enables individuals to predict accurately how others will respond to them. If patients do not appreciate, for example, that others are perceiving them as abrasive, they will not anticipate negative response. An awareness of how one is influencing others also allows the individual to make adaptive changes. It is difficult to modify abrasive conduct, for example, unless one knows in what way others are experiencing one as abrasive.

As the history is taken, the patient usually provides examples of interpersonal interactions that were unsuccessful. In discussing these relationships, patients may reveal something of their own role in contributing to such failure. If such revelations are not volunteered, patients can be asked questions such as "How did you contribute to the problem?" or "Were there aspects of your behavior or attitudes that adversely influenced the relationship?" Most patients who are not severely disturbed have some understanding of their impact on the environment. In order to gain a more objective sense of the patient's impact on others and to check the accuracy of the patient's assessment, the physician can also rely on observations of how the patient comes across during the interview (for example, is the patient angry, patronizing, or seductive?).

People manage their interpersonal environments more adaptively if they know how others influence them. Those who know that they are made angry by overly passive people may wish to avoid them, and those who know that they are likely to be subservient in the presence of authority figures may seek to regulate their confrontations with powerful others. Therapeutic change in the manner in which one responds to others is also made more likely by an awareness of one's own response pattern.

Clues to the patient's pattern of response to others can be obtained from several sources. One is the past history. More immediate estimates of the patient's awareness of these patterns can be obtained by asking about this issue directly. A useful chain of questions might be "How did you react when she snubbed you?" and "Have people treated you this way before?" and "Is this the way you usually respond to people who treat you this way?" The physician can also observe how the patient responds to him or her. It is not possible, of course, to orchestrate artificial behaviors in order to observe the patient's pattern of responsivity. What is possible, however, is to observe the patient's response to the physician's authority, personal mannerisms, or (in rare circumstances, hopefully) tardiness or annoyance. Once the physician has estimated how the patient is responding, it is relatively easy to check the accuracy with which patients perceive their responses.

The Patient's Values

The degree of importance that patients attach to material possessions, friendships, work, leisure, or political or religious ideas has a critical relationship to their illness and treatment. It is always useful to ask patients what they value. Values provide people with a sense of meaning. All human beings live with the certain knowledge that ultimately they will die, and that they will never do all the things they want to do or be all the things they want to be. In order to tolerate the limitations of their existence, they seek meaning in material possessions, work, interpersonal gratifications, or belief systems. Experiences of illness often change the way in which patients value people, work, things, or ideas. Some patients develop distorted value systems as a result of illness. Others continue to reexamine their values as they grow older and come, in time, to reject or to alter value systems that have sustained them in the past.

Values are inferred from patients' statements and from the history of their past behavior. Sophisticated patients (who are not very disturbed) can be asked directly about what is most important to them. The physician will find that discrepancies between patients' professed values and their past behavior are common. A patient who proclaims that serving others is the highest possible value may have spent his or her life doing little more than accumulating wealth. Many patients are aware of these discrepancies and, as a result, suffer a diminished self-concept. The extent of the patient's awareness of discrepancies can be estimated by asking such a question as "Do you feel you have been able to live according to your value system?"

The physician should also consider the consistency with which patients have acted on their values in relating to those closest to them. Some people who hold to altruistic values are able to exercise them in either close or distant relationships, but not in both. The most benevolent and charitable public citizen may be a tyrant at home. In contrast, the loving and unselfish family member may have no qualms about exploiting strangers.

While inquiring about values and meaningfulness, the physician may also wish to learn about how patients view the most critical issue of existence: their own mortality. Existentialists assert that fear of death and coping with the idea of death are important determinants of all psychiatric symptomatology. Whether or not this is true, patients' attitudes toward death or dying certainly influence their responses both to sickness and to treatment. With any but the most disturbed patient, it is useful to inquire about this issue. A possible series of questions that the physicians may wish to ask are "Do you ever think or worry about death?" and "What do you feel will happen to you when you die?" and "How do your thoughts about death influence your current attitudes and behavior?"

Patients' Attitudes toward Their Illness

Traditionally, patients' attitudes toward their illness are discussed under the rubric of insight. From the standpoint of both diagnosis and treatment, it is usually important to know if patients recognize that they are ill. There is much more, however, to assessing attitudes toward illness than simply determining the patient's awareness of its existence. The physician should also try to learn something about patients' moral views of their illness, their attempts to explain it, and their motivations to overcome it.

The experience of distress or disability changes patients' self-concept and their ability to cope with the environment. Many patients evaluate this change in moral terms. Patients are told repeatedly that their illness is an affliction that they had no role in creating; they may nonetheless experience their psychological symptoms as evidence of weakness of the will. They judge themselves negatively, and this moral judgment may play a role in creating the commonly observed phenomenon of their becoming depressed over being depressed or anxious about being anxious. (Other factors, such as the incapacities created by symptoms and the reactions of others, are, of course, also involved in this phenomenon.) The physician can inquire about the existence of this kind of self-judgment by asking directly how patients' symptoms have influenced their view of themselves. Questions such as "Do you ever get angry at yourself for being sick?" and "Do you get depressed after you are symptomatic?" may also be helpful. The presence of negative attitudes toward symptomatology suggests the need for therapeutic interventions designed to change the manner in which patients think about their illness.

There are other clinically relevant aspects of how patients explain illness to themselves that are nonjudgmental. From the time of Thomas Hobbes, psychologists have noted that, because each human being is more familiar with his or her own internal experiences than with anyone else's, each person tends to develop a private system for explaining their presence. This system is characterized by different degrees of emphasis on environmental, biological, or psychological variables. Environmental and biological factors are usually viewed as being outside one's control; psychological factors tend to be viewed as aspects of the will.

The physician often encounters patients who take extreme positions about the causation of their symptoms; they view their symptoms as either completely under their control or completely beyond their control. As a rule, patients who tend to view their symptoms as self-determined are described as *psychological-minded*. Psychotherapy requires that they learn how to control their behavior and attitudes. Because they take some responsibility for their symptoms, they are likely to be active and effective participants in such efforts. (Sometimes, they do this to a fault, pursuing "growth-oriented" psychotherapy for years when pharmacotherapy would help them more quickly.) Patients who regard their symptoms as stemming from sources out of their control may envision successful treatment as being dependent on some external happening, either a change in a stressful environment or some biological attenuation of their condition. These patients are less likely to be good psychotherapy candidates and are more likely to cooperate with biological and environmental interventions.

Patients' views of the cause of their symptoms can usually be determined by asking them directly about their perceptions of etiology. Other cues can be elicited during history taking, when they may attribute emotional problems to controllable or uncontrollable circumstances. The physician can learn more about these issues by asking questions such as "Was there anything you could have done to avoid this illness?" or "What can you do to make things better?" or "Do you feel there is anything you can do to change things?"

Finally, patients may vary in their motivations to get well. This is an important variable in treatment, as highly motivated patients are more cooperative in psychotherapy and in following the physician's instructions. Some patients have adapted to their symptoms and have learned to use the sick role to gratify dependency needs. Even though they may be quite miserable, they may not be highly motivated to give up the reinforcements associated with the sick behavior. Other patients may not view their symptoms, particularly their behavioral symptoms, as troubling and may not want to do much to change them. These patients are less cooperative in treatment.

In assessing motivation, the physician tries, first of all, to determine how much distress the patient is experiencing. The degree of willingness that patients have to share the extent of their suffering gives some clues to how fervently they desire relief. This information, however, is not always a reliable index of how cooperative the patient will be. Some patients complain vehemently about their suffering, insist that they will do anything to get well, and then cooperate poorly in treatment. It is also useful for the physician to assess the power of the reinforcements that the patient receives as a result of illness. These can be weighed against the patient's level of distress to obtain a very rough evaluation of motivation.

FOR FURTHER READING

Berkowitz, L. *Aggression: A social psychological analysis*. McGraw-Hill, New York, 1962.

Brenner, C. The masochistic character. *Journal of the American Psychoanalytic Association*, 7:197, 1959.

Cleckley, H. *The mask of sanity*. C. V. Mosby, St. Louis, 1950.

Grotevant, H. D., and Carlson, C. I. *Family assessment*. Guilford, New York, 1989.

Halleck, S. L. Hysterical personality traits: Psychological, social and iatrogenic determinants. *Archives of General Psychiatry*, 16:750, 1967.

Halleck, S. L. *Psychiatry and the dilemmas of crime*. Harper, New York, 1967.

Kernberg, O. F. *Borderline conditions and pathological narcissism*. Aranson, New York, 1975.

Kernberg, O. F. *Severe personality disorders: Psychotherapeutic strategies*. Yale University Press, New Haven, CT, 1989.

Knight, R. P. Borderline states. *Bulletin of the Menninger Clinic*, 7:1, 1953.

Kohut, H., and Wolff, E. S. The disorders of the self and their treatment: An outline. *International Journal of Psychoanalysis*, 59:413, 1978.

Lion, J. R. (Ed.) *Personality disorders: Diagnosis and management*, (2nd ed.). Williams & Wilkins, Baltimore, 1981.

Menninger, K. A. *The vital balance*. Viking Press, New York, 1963.

Menninger, W. W. The chronically mentally ill. In *Comprehensive textbook of psychiatry*, *Vol. 5*, H. I. Kaplan and B. J. Sadock (Eds.). Williams & Wilkins, Baltimore, 1989.

Millon, T. Disorders of personality. *DSM-III–Axis-II*. Wiley, New York, 1981.

Salzman, L. Paranoid states: Theory and treatment. *Archives of General Psychiatry*, 2:107, 1960.

Salzman, L. *The obsessive personality*. Science House, New York, 1968.

Speck, R., and Attneave, C. In *Network therapy: The book of family therapy*, A. Farber, M. Mendelsohn, and A. Napier, (Eds.). Errenson, New York, 1972.

Stone, M. *The borderline syndromes*. McGraw-Hill, New York, 1980.

Vaillant, G. E. *Adaptation to life*. Little, Brown, Boston, 1977.

Wallerstein, R. *Forty-two lives in treatment*. Guilford, New York, 1986.

CHAPTER SIX

The Mental Status Examination

The mental status examination is a study of the patient's behavior and experience, primarily within the environment of the examination itself. Therefore, it deals mainly with the present, not the past. Because it consists of time-limited observations, it is ordinarily viewed as a cross-sectional rather than a longitudinal view of the patient's behavior and experience.

Modern writers have referred to the mental status examination as the psychiatric analogue of the physical examination in other branches of medicine. Although this view is not precisely accurate, like the physical examination the mental status examination does consist of efforts both to assess the patient's behavior and experience objectively and to determine the patient's responses to various tests of current organismic functioning. When systematically conceptualized and recorded, the mental status examination is an instrument that helps the psychiatrist to determine the presence of many and, in some cases, most of the criteria for major psychiatric disorders.

The mental status examination is most useful when it is based on a phenomenological approach. This requires that psychopathology be observed and accurately described, and that an emphasis on explanation be postponed. Explanations of abnormal psychiatric findings may be essential for treatment planning, but explanatory systems should not be allowed to influence a phase of evaluation that requires objective observation. The reason is that a premature commitment to theoretical notions about causation may encourage the clinician to overvalue data that confirm certain hypotheses and to ignore data that do not.

While the mental status examination is an assessment of current mental functioning, it is usually impossible to make this assessment without learning a little about the patient's past. Delusional beliefs or hallucinations, for example, may not exist at the precise moment of the examination but may be a significant aspect of the patient's current functioning. A patient who says that Martians follow him all day long, but that they leave him alone when the doctor is around, should be described as having a delusional perception (a delusion based on a hallucinatory experience); this is true even if that experience is not manifested during the interview. A person can report hearing strange howling voices whenever evening approaches; however, she might not be hallucinating in this fashion when examined in the morning. Even though the account of these symptoms is derived from history taking rather than direct observation, it would be confusing and inconvenient to report them as part of the history rather than as an aspect of the mental status examination.

It is also important to emphasize that the mental status examination is not a discrete aspect of the total examination; it does not begin at some distinct point in time after the history has been taken. As a rule, the most critical aspects of patients' motor and verbal behavior as well as of their experiences are revealed in the process of taking the history. There may be a particular point in the evaluation where certain aspects of perceiving and thinking are formally tested, but this is only one aspect of the mental status examination.

It is appropriate once again to emphasize the importance of history taking, in this instance as an essential aspect of the mental status examination. Some hospital settings currently allow social workers to relieve the doctor of the "burden" of history taking and require that the physician report only the mental status examination. This is a deplorable means of saving the doctor's time. It is unlikely that an accurate mental status examination can be done when the physician has no opportunity to observe how patients discuss their life stories.

Before getting into the main body of this chapter, I would also like to take issue with that school of psychiatry that teaches that the *content* of psychopathology as opposed to the *form* is rarely important in the mental status examination. Those who hold to this view argue that the mental impairments associated with mental disorders have a consistent form, and that their form can be fully evaluated without considering their content. They view content as environmentally (usually culturally) determined and not relevant to the process of diagnosing the diseases of individuals. Such an approach might make sense if the doctor never did anything but diagnose for the sake of categorization. Once treatment or any type of intervention is considered, however, the content of the patient's thoughts and feelings particularly as they relate to the environment is critical. It is not sufficient merely to note that a patient has voiced murderous thoughts toward others. Knowing which individuals have been threatened, the reasons that the patient gives to justify such thoughts, and the manner in which he or she plans to deal with them are of utmost importance. They matter both to the clinician who wishes to help the patient and to those who may be harmed by the patient. The content of delusional ideas is equally important. A patient who has a delusional belief that he or she will soon experience a painful death may be at high risk of committing suicide. A patient who believes that certain people are planning to hurt him or her may strike out at them. Sometimes even the content of a delusion can provide clues to problems of stress or conflict. Thus, the patient who expresses a false belief that his wife is poisoning him may have "selected" that particular delusion because he is experiencing severe conflict in his marriage.

WHAT MATERIAL SHOULD BE COVERED IN A MENTAL STATUS EXAMINATION, AND HOW SHOULD IT BE RECORDED?

The approach here is traditional. This means the examiner should seek information about the patient's general appearance, motor behavior, emotional state, form and content of thought, perception, and cognitive functioning. Although each of these areas must be assessed, the amount of information recorded will be determined by the evaluator's decisions about which data are most relevant. Obviously, all pathological findings should be recorded. Some aspects of the mental status examination such as the patient's general appearance, motor behavior, or affect should be commented on because diagnostic information is generally provided merely by describing them. It is also useful to record something about normal mental processes, particularly the results of tests of cognition, so that subsequent treaters can compare these data with their more current evaluation. In thinking about the organization of the mental status examination, it is useful to consider the answers to the questions What? Why? How? What should the examiner evaluate? Why should it be evaluated? And how should the evaluation be done?

WHAT ASPECTS OF THE PATIENT'S GENERAL APPEARANCE SHOULD BE EVALUATED?

The physician should note or evaluate the patient's age, race, sex, body type, state of consciousness, manner, nutrition, health, and personal hygiene. The reasons for observing each of these factors are as follows:

Age

Various mental as well as physical disorders are more likely to be manifested at different ages. Depression and dementia are more common in the elderly. Schizophrenia and manic-depressive disorders are likely to develop in early adulthood. The patient's age also gives clues to various developmental problems that the patient may be encountering. Knowledge of the patient's age may also help the clinician assess the risk of the patient's being violent. Most violent acts are committed by late adolescents and young adults. Finally, those who look older than their stated age may have experienced considerable illness or chronic suffering.

Race

Some physical illnesses, such as hypertension, sickle-cell anemia, or skin cancer, may be associated with race. Race and sometimes ethnicity also provide statistical clues to the patient's socioeconomic status and the nature of his or her previous life experience. A black patient in the United States, for example, is much more likely than a white patient to have experienced poverty, discrimination, poor health care, and violence. These experiences have a major influence on mental and physical development and are a factor in causing or complicating mental disorders.

Sex

Some mental disorders, such as histrionic personality disorder or depression, are more common in females, and others, such as antisocial personality disorder or most of the impulse control disorders, are more common in males. Many physical disorders are also gender-related. Whether gender differences in the prevalence of mental disorders are environmentally or biologically determined, the patient's sex tells the clinician something about the statistical likelihood of his or her having various mental disorders. The physician can also anticipate that the patient's social conditioning based on sex-role assignments will have influenced his or her personality development, how the patient deals with symptoms, and how the individual will respond to treatment.

Body Type and Characteristics

The patient's general bone and muscle structure (ectomorphic, mesomorphic, or endomorphic) may be associated with a greater propensity to develop a variety of mental and perhaps physical illnesses. Body characteristics such as obesity, obvious disfigurements, or unusual patterns of hair distribution give clues to physical impairments. Such anomalous physical traits are developmental idiosyncrasies that may have caused the patient to experience considerable trauma as a child.

Obviously, abnormal physical characteristics such as jaundice or hirsutism have direct diagnostic significance.

State of Consciousness

Patients who have difficulty in staying awake or in listening to or responding to the examiner's questions are displaying a reduced level of consciousness; this is a diagnostic sign of delirium. The finding of diminished alertness is especially critical in elderly patients, who may also appear confused, perplexed, agitated, and restless. More severe alterations in consciousness, such as semicoma (in which the patient responds only if shaken or shouted at) or coma (in which the patient is unresponsive even to painful stimuli), are generally associated with known and usually severe organic disorders. Patients with catatonia may also appear to have diminished levels of alertness.

Manner

Evaluating patients' manner of approaching the examination—whether they are cooperative, friendly, passive, ingratiating, seductive, obsequious, or guarded—requires judgment and inference as well as observation. Although observation of the patient's manner may not provide direct diagnostic clues, it often helps the clinician confirm the presence of certain personality traits. Sometimes, it helps the clinician to gauge the accuracy of the patient's communications. The patient's manner also provides clues to the possibility of imminent violence. Surly, suspicious, restless, and uncooperative patients have a higher potential of being violent and should be interviewed in a tactful and usually nonchallenging manner.

Personal Hygiene

Poor personal hygiene may be associated with extreme poverty or the rejection of conventional societal standards, but it may also be a sign of serious mental or physical illness. Depressed or psychotic patients may be too fatigued, preoccupied, or perplexed to care adequately for their personal needs. During the deteriorating stage of their disorder, alcoholics are notoriously likely to appear in emergency rooms in an unkempt state.

Having observed the patient's sex and race at that first meeting, the physician usually makes a rough assessment of the patient's age at the same time. It is always useful, however, to make a direct inquiry about the patient's age and to record it precisely. Body types and bodily characteristics, personal hygiene, state of consciousness, and manner are all evaluated as the interview and the process of history taking progress. The patient's state of consciousness may not be immediately apparent, but during the interview, fluctuations in alertness generally become obvious. It is only as the interview progresses, and as underlying attitudes become manifest (or can be inferred), that judgments about the patient's manner are possible.

WHAT ISSUES DOES THE PHYSICIAN CONSIDER IN EVALUATING THE PATIENT'S MOTOR BEHAVIOR?

The physician routinely observes the patient's gait and looks for abnormal movements that appear to be either voluntary or involuntary. Patients may show various unsteady and unsymmetrical gaits as well as a lack of coordination of arm and leg movements. Some patients demonstrate continuous smooth or jerky movements (referred to respectively as *athetosis* or *chorea*). Involuntary movements of the tongue, mouth, facial muscles, and shoulders are common in patients who have been taking neuroleptics for many months or years (tardive dyskinesia). Still other patients will show movements (tics) such as blinking, grunting, sniffing, rubbing of body parts, or twitching. These appear to be under voluntary control but are not experienced as voluntary to patients who find them distinctly troubling.

The extent of the patient's movement should also be observed. Some patients appear unable to sit still; they pace, wring their hands, bite their nails, twist their hair, and constantly shift positions. Such constant movement that is not goal-directed is described as *agitation*. Patients may demonstrate a marked increase in the rate of motor behavior that is more goal-directed. These patients, usually seen in the hospital setting, may move from task to task in rapid succession (e.g., from cleaning, to writing, to rearranging their personal belongings). This behavior is referred to as *hyperactivity* and, when extreme, as *excitement*.

Other patients show diminished activity or hyperactivity. They may sit in the same position for hours and barely respond to the examiner's inquiries. At the extreme, hypoactivity may be characterized by complete muteness and even by unresponsiveness to painful stimuli. This condition is called *stupor*.

Other patients position their body parts in inappropriate or odd ways. This is described as *posturing*. If patients retain odd postures for long periods of time, they are described as having *catalepsy*. Patients who show posturing and catalepsy are called *catatonic*. They may also show bizarre motor signs, such as mimicking the examiner's movements (echopraxia) or providing only slow resistance when the examiner places their extremities in odd positions (waxy flexibility).

Abnormal gaits (which will not be described here) may be indicative of extrapyramidal, frontal lobe, or cerebellar dysfunction. Asymmetry in gait suggests previous orthopedic or neurological injury. Jerky or smooth movements that appear to be involuntary suggest extrapyramidal disease, and the observation of jerky movements often tips the examiner off to the presence of Huntington's chorea.

Agitated patients are usually very anxious and/or depressed. Their agitation may be viewed as a motoric expression of a painful emotional state. Agitation is also a major clue to impending violence. The clinician must be especially careful in dealing with the patient who paces about the room and who appears intensely distraught. In assessing agitated behavior, the clinician should be aware that patients who take neuroleptic drugs may show symptoms of motor restlessness that are quite similar to agitated behavior (akathisia). Their motor restlessness, however, is a side effect of the medication and may not be associated with painful emotional states.

Hypoactive patients may be showing signs of physical illness or may be depressed. Here, too, the physician must be aware of the effect of psychotropic drugs. Neuroleptic agents can produce a stiffness and slowness of activity (akinesia) that may be unrelated to emotional states.

Patients who show excitement, stupor, posturing, catalepsy, and waxy flexibility have a syndrome called *catatonia* (sometimes viewed as a form of schizophrenia). This is usually treated effectively with electric convulsive treatment.

Motor behavior is assessed primarily by observation. The patient's gait can be observed as the physician walks with the patient to the examining room. Other disorders of movement are noted as the history is taken. Patients can sometimes be asked to try to control certain movements to test the degree to which such movements are voluntary. More sophisticated evaluations of localized motoric dysfunctions are obtained by doing a neurological examination.

WHAT ISSUES DOES THE PHYSICIAN CONSIDER IN ASSESSING THE PATIENT'S EMOTIONAL STATE?

The sense of well-being or of suffering that patients experience is a function of their emotional state, that is, how they feel. When clinicians assess emotionality, they are sometimes interested in states of increased feelings of well-being, but for the most part, they are simply trying to determine the nature and degree of the patient's suffering. In many ways, in psychiatry, the evaluation of emotion is similar to the evaluation of pain in other branches of medicine. Whenever the patient complains of an unpleasant emotion (such as anxiety or sadness), the clinician will want to know how that emotion is experienced, exactly what it feels like, how severe it is perceived to be, how long it lasts, what brings it on, and what relieves it.

Although students of psychiatry are generally urged to evaluate emotionality as part of the mental status examination (a cross-sectional evaluation), it is difficult to learn much about emotionality without considering the patient's recent history. The actual psychiatric interview creates a unique environment for patients, and the feelings they experience during the interview are often different from those they may have experienced only minutes before. If a patient states that, for several hours preceding the interview, he has been continuously anxious or sad but happens to feel better during the interview, it is more convenient to describe his painful emotionality as part of the mental status examination as well as part of the history.

Assessing the patient's emotional life also requires the clinician to consider the relationship of emotions to other mental functions. Aberrations of either thinking or behavior are likely to have an adverse influence on how the patient feels. The patient who experiences self-critical thoughts generally feels worse. So does the patient who behaves poorly and experiences a sense of loss of control, or who fears retaliation from others.

Another critical issue in assessing emotionality is the reliability of patient's descriptions of their experiences. Some patients cannot describe their feelings very well, and often, they describe them inaccurately. Here, the clinician must use empathic skills and ask questions such as "Does it feel as if you want to cry?" or "Do you feel a sense of impending doom?" to help patients identify the exact nature of their emotions.

Most psychiatric texts describe the emotional life of the patient by using two separate terms: *affect* and *mood*. *Affect* sometimes refers to the emotional tone associated with behavior and other mental processes over a period of time, either the length of the interview or, by history, an arbitrary length of time (hours, days, or weeks). The term *mood* is used to refer to the patient's immediate emotional state. In this nomenclature, mood becomes a part of the patient's affect, the part that is observed at any given moment. It should be noted that some authors reverse this usage. The DSM-III-R uses the term *mood* to describe a prolonged emotional state. Other authors use the term *mood* to refer to the patient's reported feeling state and the term *affect* to refer to the clinician's inference about the patient's emotionality (as judged by the patient's facial expressions and other nonverbal cues).

The inconsistent use of terms to describe various aspects of emotionality can be confusing to the student. For this reason it is sometimes wise to avoid the use of terms like *mood* or *affect*, and to simply focus on description of the patient's emotional state over time. The physician should be concerned about precisely defining the major emotional state or states the patient appears to be experiencing during the interview or describes having recently experienced. As emotional states change, the physician will be interested in noting how they change, how frequently new states appear, and how such changes take place.

The major emotions that patients experience are sadness, happiness, anxiety, anger, and apathy. Each of these feeling states may have varying degrees of intensity. A sad patient may feel slightly "down" or hopelessly depressed. A happy patient may feel comfortable, moderately elated, or euphoric. An anxious patient may feel tense, jittery, or panicky. Anger may vary from irritability to rage; apathy from mild lack of interest to complete withdrawal. There are many adjectives that the clinician can use to describe the intensity of the patient's immediate emotional state. It is helpful to seek the most precise adjective and, when this is not possible, to try to grade the intensity of the patient's emotionality by using terms such as *mild, moderate,* or *severe.*

When emotions are evaluated over time, the clinician is concerned about their range, their variety, the manner in which they change, and their rate of change. Some patients may demonstrate only a single emotional state, such as sadness, during the entire interview; the range of their emotionality is then described as *constricted.* Other patients may have rapid variations in emotional states, sometimes shifting from sadness to euphoria for no apparent reason. They are described as having *labile emotionality.* Patients who show little range or intensity of emotional states over time and who appear to be primarily apathetic are described as *emotionally blunted.*

The clinician is also interested in judging whether the emotional state that patients experience at any given moment is logically related to the content of their verbal statements. Patients who laugh when describing a tragedy are demonstrating an incongruity between the content of their thoughts and their apparent emotionality. Although such an incongruity may have many clinical meanings, the emotionality is best described as *inappropriate.*

Patients experience unpleasant emotional states as symptoms, and these symptoms are elements of major diagnostic categories. The observations of sadness, elation, or anxiety suggest the diagnosis of an affective or an anxiety disorder. Apathy, particularly if it is associated with emotional blunting (a diminution in the range and intensity of emotional states), is often a symptom of schizophrenia. Observation of the emotion of anger has practical relevance for the safety of the interviewer; moreover, it may provide support for diagnoses of affective disorder or personality disorder. The absence of a wide range of emotionality during the interview suggests that the patient is severely disturbed. Lability of emotional state, particularly if unrelated to the content of what is being discussed, suggests the presence of a psychotic disorder, either an organic brain disorder, a manic disorder, or a schizophrenic disorder.

Aside from its diagnostic significance, observation of the patient's emotional state will influence the manner in which the evaluator conducts the interview. If the patient is angry and agitated, the evaluator must seek ways of tempering this emotion for the sake of protecting both himself or herself and the patient. With any patient, the evaluator tries to fine-tune questions so that they are relevant to the patient's emotional state. Questions that seem to ignore the seriousness of the patient's emotional distress may appear to the patient to be inappropriate. In dealing with depressed patients, for example, it is not helpful to ask about feelings of elation until the exact nature of their depressed feelings have been explored.

In evaluating emotionality, the physician's major problem is trying to identify a private experience precisely. One begins by asking the patient to describe the experience. One then may try to help the patient be more detailed and precise by suggesting descriptive adjectives (e.g., *frightening, unbearable*, or *hopeless*) or sometimes similes or metaphors ("Is it as if you are being engulfed by a dark cloud?" or "Do you feel you will lose control?").

Despite these efforts, the patient may not be very accurate, and the physician will then want more objective data. Observation of the patient's general appearances and motor behavior helps a little. Patients who say they feel depressed, look sad, and are hypoactive are probably reporting their feelings accurately. Patients who complain of anxiety, show facial expressions of fear, and are hyperactive are also likely to be accurate. If patients are mute or communicate little, their emotionality must be inferred largely on the basis of recent history, general appearance, and motor behavior. The patient's reporting of associated symptomatology will also help the physician assess the accuracy of reported emotionality. If recent behavior (e.g., insomnia, anorexia, or withdrawal from activities) is consistent with a diagnosis of depression, and the patient reports emotions of extreme sadness, the patient's reporting is likely to be accurate. Finally, the content of patients' thoughts may help in understanding their feelings. For most patients, feelings and thoughts tend to parallel one another. Ordinarily, depressed patients report thoughts that revolve around guilt, loss, and hopelessness. Elated patients talk about grandiose ideas. And anxious patients discuss their fears. It is the congruency of the data that suggests that the patient is reporting feelings accurately. If emotionality and verbal content appear to be unrelated, the accuracy of the patient's reporting must be questioned, and the presence of a psychotic process should be suspected.

WHAT GENERAL ISSUES ARE INVOLVED
IN ASSESSING THE PATIENT'S THINKING?

No one can ever know the exact content and form of another person's thinking, and, in effect, the clinician evaluates thinking primarily by studying the content and form of the patient's communications. Thinking can also be assessed by asking patients questions that test their ability to perform certain thought functions. This type of assessment is discussed in more detail in a later section that deals with cognitive functions.

The form and content of thought are highly responsive to environmental cues. As we go through a waking day, an hour, or even a minute, our thoughts and our ability to communicate them are influenced by where we are, who we are with, and what we are trying to do. The psychiatric interview creates a new environment, which patients perceive as providing various degrees of stress or support. During the course of a single interview, however, even this environment does not remain constant. As the nature of the patient's environment (including the interview environment) changes, the physician should, therefore, anticipate fluctuations in the form and content of the patient's thinking.

WHAT VARIATIONS IN THE FORM OF COMMUNICATION
DOES THE PHYSICIAN STUDY?

From the beginning of the interview, the clinician will note that some patients vary from the norm in their rate of speech. Others use language in an idiosyncratic manner. Still others do not communicate in a manner that is logical or coherent enough to be understandable. The observation of any of these variations in the form of communication suggests a disorder in thinking. Although not pathognomonic of any particular illness, each variation in speech provides clues to the possible existence of certain psychiatric disorders.

Some patients speak very slowly. This slow speech may reflect cultural patterns, personality traits, extreme cautiousness, or impaired ability to think at a normal rate. Patients who are depressed may speak slowly because they think slowly. This phenomenon may also characterize patients who have altered states of consciousness, such as stupor. Patients with organic brain disease may have difficulty in remembering all of the words in their vocabulary; the slowness they demonstrate is related to a struggle to recall the right words.

Many patients speak rapidly, a behavior that may reflect cultural patterns or personality traits. Some patients speak rapidly only when extremely anxious; such patients can usually slow down their rate of speech when asked to do so. Manic patients, on the other hand, speak very rapidly and seem unable to control the rate. They may talk continuously as though pressured to do so. Often, they acknowledge that their thoughts are racing. In its extreme form, the rapid speech of manic patients may lose logic or coherence. Their associations are not connected in a way that is understandable to others, and they jump from topic to topic for reasons that are unclear to the observer. When these patients recover, they usually ascribe their communication disorder to a condition in which they were thinking so rapidly that they could not relate one thought to another. Or they recall that they could not avoid having their thoughts constantly altered by environmental cues. The rapid rate of thinking and/or distractibility make it difficult for such patients to complete the presentation of the ideas or goals they originally wished to express. To the observer it appears that the goal of their communication is not reached.

Some patients use language idiosyncratically. They may create words that do not exist in the dictionary, such as "I lost my biodogens," and use them as substitutes for conventional words (neologisms). Or they may use unconventional and approximate terms such as *transportation device* to describe an automobile (word approximation). It is not always clear whether this use of deviant language is a deliberate attempt not to communicate clearly or a manifestation of an inability to use conventional language. Most of the time, it is the latter. Neologisms and word approximations are commonly seen in patients with schizophrenic and organic brain disorders. It is also true, however, that sometimes relatively normal people have trouble thinking of commonly used words and use less than precise language to convey their thoughts.

Some patients tend to repeat certain words or phrases, particularly at the end of a thought sequence (e.g., "I want to go out—out—out"). This is called *verbigeration* and may be associated with catatonia. Other patients insert stock words in their sentences repeatedly, even when these words do not enhance the meaning of communication. This language deviation may be culturally determined (the current useless but frequently repeated phrase is "you know"), but if the patient continually repeats phrases in a nonconventional manner, we usually describe this type of speech as *perseverative*. Repetitive use of stock phrases is often associated with organic brain syndromes.

A major class of disorders of communication occurs when patients speak at a normal rate and use conventional language but do not present their ideas clearly or understandably. The commonest of these problems involves communication in which words or phrases do not seem to be meaningfully connected. When connections between associations cannot be ascertained, we describe the patient as having *loosened associations*. There are varying degrees of severity of loosening of associations.

When individual words seem unrelated, we call such loosening *word salad*. When phrases or sentences are unrelated, we describe the communication and thinking as *fragmented*. Loosening of associations may be seen in any psychotic disorder, including manic-depressive illness, schizophrenia, or organic brain syndromes.

Another frequent form of deviant communication is characterized by an indirect and usually prolonged expression of a particular idea. These patients may reach their goal, but they do so circuitously, interspersing their sentences with ideas that are not essential to their central theme. This form of communication disorder is called *circumstantiality* and is seen in a variety of major and minor mental disorders. In its less extreme form, it may be seen in the elderly and in obsessive patients who wish to keep the examiner's attention or who are concerned that every single detail related to their ideas be presented. In the elderly, circumstantiality is sometimes viewed as a sign of organicity, but this is not necessarily true. The elderly who are often alone and are not used to having an audience may intersperse their talk with digressions in order to keep the listener tuned in longer. Obsessive patients become circumstantial when they are concerned with the possibility that they may leave out some important detail. Extreme examples of circumstantiality are also seen in manic-depressive disorders and organic brain disease. Whatever the cause of circumstantial communication, it has a distinct impact on the interviewer, who usually feels uncomfortably captured by the patient's communication, has difficulty in following it, and quickly becomes restless and bored.

There are other forms of dissolution of logic or lack of continuity of the patient's expressed ideas. *Tangential communication* refers to speech in which, initially, the ideas seem related, but in which patients go off in unrelated directions and never reach their goal. In its mildest form, the tangent may have some detectable relationship to the idea the patient was originally expressing. This can sometimes occur in patients who are preoccupied with their problems and are not concentrating on connections and logic. In other situations, connections may not be discernable. Here, the unrelatedness of communication is so severe that the patient's speech is spoken of as *fragmented* (words, phrases, or sentences are not meaningfully connected), *rambling* (fragmented and not goal-directed), or *derailed* (suddenly switching to a totally new line of thought). The term *nonsequitur* (which means "not to follow") is ordinarily used to describe responses that are not relevant to the questions. An example is a patient who, when asked "How old are you?," replies, "The sun will set at 8 P.M. tonight." Patients who respond to questions with nonsequiturs often (but not always) show other manifestations of disturbed speech, such as fragmentation, rambling, tangentiality, or derailment. The major disruptions in the logical links of associations tend to be found in the more severe psychiatric disorders, especially those of psychotic degree, such as manic-depressive illness, schizophrenia, or organic brain syndrome.

There are several other deviations in the form of communication that are important. Manic patients sometimes seem to make their associations by the sound of words rather than by the meaning of words ("I went to the house, the mouse and a louse bit me"). These are called *clang associations*. Schizophrenic patients and patients with organic brain syndromes may suddenly appear to lose their train of thought. At times, of course, this happens to all of us, but we are aware of it and usually make some attempt to apologize for it or to cover it up. When patients lose their train of thought, appear not to be aware of it, and go on talking about an unrelated subject, we call this phenomenon *blocking*. Manic patients sometimes show combinations of fragmented and circumstantial communications with deviations from logical links apparently related to environmental cues, for example, "I'm hungry. Who are you? That's a pretty blue suit you're wearing; I love blue sky; I love blueberry pie. When do we eat?" This phenomenon is referred to as *flight of ideas*.

It is important for the interviewer to keep in mind that all of the above forms of communication are made worse by the patient's anxiety. A skillful interviewer can often diminish the severity of the patient's disturbed communication. Even the beginner will notice that, as the interview progresses, some patients become more comfortable and communicate more effectively. The degree to which patients communicate better as they feel more at ease is, of course, related to the type of disturbance they have. Nonpsychotic patients improve markedly. As a rule, even schizophrenic patients can do much better when they are calmer. The only group of patients who may show little improvement are those who are severely organically impaired.

WHAT ASPECTS OF THE CONTENT OF THE PATIENT'S THOUGHTS DOES THE PHYSICIAN ASSESS?

In the nature of things, the psychiatric evaluator is interested primarily in abnormal thought content. However, it is useful to observe and describe any recurrent themes (sometimes called *preoccupations*) to which the patient repeatedly returns during the course of history taking. Such preoccupations matter whether they appear to be abnormal or not. Some patients focus on specific life problems or on their symptoms. These preoccupations can be considered disturbances in the content of thought, even if they are appropriate to the patient's life situation. Although most texts on the mental status examination do not recommend noting these findings, they may be highly relevant to the treatment of the patient. Awareness of the patient's preoccupations provides clues to what issues may have to be resolved before the patient can feel better.

Some patients are preoccupied with unpleasant thoughts unrelated to any obvious life problems. Patients experience these preoccupations as symptoms. Persistent and unwanted thoughts (sometimes called *obsessions*) may be experienced as intrusive. The patient is aware that they are senseless but feels unable to stop them. Patients troubled by obsessional thinking often experience thoughts of doing harm to themselves or others; as a rule, this type of thinking is not associated with suicidal or violent behavior. Obviously, it is important to distinguish this pattern from deliberate consideration of or active planning for a suicidal or violent act, which serves as a predictor of such behavior.

There are patients who perceive their obsessive thoughts as blasphemous. This perception can create powerful experiences of anxiety in highly moralistic or religious individuals. Still other patients are obsessed with being harmed by natural phenomena or supernatural forces. They may unrealistically fear bacterial contamination or supernatural disaster. These patients may feel compelled to perform some ritualistic act such as hand washing or to engage in a meaningless motor movement, either of which is designed to neutralize the painful emotional state associated with their thinking.

Although phobias are usually thought of as behavioral disorders, they are also associated with characteristic patterns of thinking. Phobic patients are often preoccupied with structuring their lives so as to avoid a feared object or situation. Even when they are successful, they may still devote a great deal of their waking life to thinking and worrying about situations in which they may not be able to avoid the feared object.

Hypochondriacal preoccupation is generally associated with the unpleasant emotional states of fear and anxiety. In describing the current manifestations of this symptom, the evaluator should note how such patients regard medical evidence that they do not have a serious illness, and how steadfastly they hold to the belief that they are ill in the face of such a confrontation. It is difficult, at times, to determine when the patient's hypochondriasis is so irrational as to be considered delusional.

Delusions are false beliefs that the patient retains even in the face of incontrovertible evidence to the contrary. (A more flippant definition of *delusion* is "a false belief outside the area of religion or politics.") There is no clear dividing line between delusional thinking and the kind of false beliefs associated with obsessive, compulsive, phobic, or hypochondriacal symptoms. Phobic patients, after all, believe that nondangerous objects or situations are dangerous, compulsive patients appear to believe that performing certain senseless acts such as decontaminating

their mail protects them from illness, and hypochondriacs insist that
they are sick even if every medical test assures them that they are well.
False beliefs associated with phobias, compulsions, or hypochondriasis
are not usually considered delusional, both because the patient usually
has at least some appreciation of their irrationality (more so in the case of
the phobic or the compulsive than the hypochondriac), and because they
are not usually associated with other symptoms of serious mental
disorder.

Ordinarily, true delusional thinking is viewed as evidence of a major psychiatric disorder. When it is present, several other mental functions are also likely to be impaired. Some patients, however, maintain
false beliefs only about isolated aspects of their lives; such individuals
appear to function very well in all other ways. I once treated a distinguished professor who believed I was hypnotizing him. When he left
treatment to take a position as vice-president of a major university, he
still voiced concerns that I had hypnotized him; nonetheless, in every
other aspect of his life he was functioning very well.

There are patients whose delusions are more bizarre and are associated with greater dysfunction. In dealing with such an individual, the
evaluator should note how the content of the delusion is related to the
patient's mood. Depressed patients may develop delusions that are congruent with their mood and that reflect unrealistic beliefs about their
down-trodden status. They may volunteer statements such as "I am
doomed," "I am the cause of all evil in the world," "I have a fatal illness,"
"My body is rotting," "I am doomed to poverty," or "I am being punished by devils because I have committed the ultimate sin." Sometimes,
depressed patients do not adhere firmly to their self-deprecatory ideas
and appear to be stating them primarily to convince others of the degree
of their suffering. In other instances, however, depressed patients firmly
adhere to irrational ideas of their own worthlessness.

The delusions of manic patients are likely to be expansive and grandiose. Statements such as "I am all-powerful," "I am the son of God," or
"I am king of all the universe" are common. The patient usually believes
these statements, but the tenacity of the belief system is variable. In the
early stages of mania, patients can be "talked out of" grandiose ideas by
an appeal to their reason. In later stages, this may be impossible.

Certainly, delusional ideas are related to mood and tend to come
and go as the patient's emotional state changes. As a rule, such ideas are
discussed spontaneously by patients. If severely depressed patients do
not bring up delusional material, it is useful to ask them, "How do you
account for your misfortune and misery?" If delusional material is present, the response to this question usually brings it out. Manic patients
who do not spontaneously discuss delusional ideas can be asked if their
feeling of well-being is associated with any type of special power.

Once cued, they are usually more than willing to discuss their expansive ideas.

Delusions may also appear to be related to other psychological phenomena, such as hallucinations or memory loss. If a patient hears a voice telling him that he is the son of God, he may well conclude that he is Jesus Christ. It is unlikely that the process of delusion formation as a result of hallucination is this simple. Conceivably, the presence of delusions also increases the likelihood of the patient's having false perceptions that reinforce the false belief. The experience of memory loss is extremely painful for most people, and one way of dealing with it is to deny that it is happening. Patients who repeatedly fail to recall where they have put things may come to believe that others are actually stealing them.

The term *primary delusion* has been reserved for those false ideas that cannot be explained on the basis of other psychological processes. Delusions that can be related to abnormal affective states, hallucinations, or impaired memory are sometimes called *secondary delusions*. The content of primary delusions is likely to reflect ideas of persecution. These ideas are often related to some environmental event that is not unusual but that patients interpret as having some special meaning for them (called a *delusional perception*). Examples of these kinds of phenomena are "She always looks nervous when I come into the room; that's how I know she's part of the plot to destroy me," and "Every time he goes into the boss's office, I know they're trying to figure out how to turn me in to the FBI."

Other types of delusional phenomena are difficult to classify either as primary or as secondarily related to hallucinatory experiences. These include such symptoms as thought broadcasting, experience of influence, or experience of alienation. *Thought broadcasting* refers to patients' reporting that their own thoughts escape from their head as they occur and that they can be heard aloud by others. It is difficult to know if these patients simply believe this, or if their belief is reinforced by some type of hallucinatory experience. *Experiences of influence* refers to patients' reporting that their feelings and thoughts are controlled by some external agency. Sometimes, this external agency is perceived as taking away or withdrawing the patient's thoughts. In experiences of alienation, patients state that their thoughts and feelings are not their own but someone else's. In the experience of both influence and alienation, it is difficult to know whether patients are having a false perception and what they are actually experiencing. Because these symptoms are usually associated with the diagnosis of schizophrenia, aside from the wonderment they elicit in any curious clinician, they may also have diagnostic relevance.

Highly disturbed patients frequently discuss delusional material openly. Less disturbed patients, whose perception of reality is some-what better, may sense that other people will view their beliefs as evidence of "craziness" and will be reluctant to acknowledge them. The best way to learn about the existence of delusions that the patient is reluctant to discuss is, of course, to gain enough rapport and trust so that patients are willing to overcome their reluctance. This process may take considerable time, however, and the clinician may need to know about delusional material not only to make a diagnosis, but also to assess the patient's potential dangerousness and treatment needs.

Usually, the clinician has cause to suspect the possibility of delusional thinking, especially when patients have behaved strangely and are showing other signs of emotional distress or difficulty in organizing their thoughts. Sometimes, these patients will discuss delusional ideas if they are directly asked such questions as "Are others treating you badly?" or "Do you feel that people are trying to influence you in some secret or unfriendly way?" A better technique is to focus on patients' explanations of their own abnormal behavior and experiences or on their explanations of the behavior of others. In one sense, delusions can be viewed as explanatory devices. They are means that the patient uses to account for abnormal phenomena (such as an altered mood or hallucinations) or to rationalize inadequacies in thinking or performance. If careful inquiries are made about how patients try to explain what is happening to them and to their "world," they may be willing to reveal the presence of delusional explanations.

Inquiries should also be made about how the patient explains unusual phenomena, such as episodes of violence, withdrawal, altered mood, or memory lapse. It is especially important to inquire about what the patient was thinking both before and during episodes of abnormal behavior. Such an inquiry may, of course, produce a rational explanation. More disturbed patients, however, may be unable to come up with any explanation at all or may reveal that their behavior was associated with bizarre or clearly false ideas. Asking for explanations about the behavior of others may elicit similar data. Questions such as "Why do you suppose your wife left you then?" or "What do you think your boss was thinking about when he asked you to take the day off?" or "Why do you think your co-workers are so competitive?" or "Do you wonder why he stopped dating you?" help to elicit evidences of delusions if they exist.

Any statement that a patient makes that appears to be delusional should be fleshed out in detail. Not only should patients be asked to say more about their beliefs, but as noted in Chapter Three, it is also necessary to ask them how they know their beliefs are true, whether they ever doubt them, whether they think others will think their beliefs are bizarre, and whether they can accept alternative explanations for the phenomena.

HOW DOES THE PHYSICIAN EVALUATE THOUGHTS
ABOUT SUICIDE AND VIOLENCE TOWARD OTHERS?

Some patients have frequent thoughts of doing violence to themselves and/or others but are not motivated to act on these thoughts.
Frequently, these thoughts are frightening to the patient. At times, however, they may not be frightening and may even be soothing. A patient
may be comforted by fantasizing revenge against an enemy or by thinking about how sorely he or she will be missed by loved ones when dead.

Although the clinician is always interested in the content of the
patient's thoughts about violence, it is most important to assess the
patient's motivations to do violence. *Motivation* can be defined as the
force or energy that induces an individual to seek a goal or to satisfy a
need or wish. It is manifested by strong emotions as well as thoughts. In
practice, there are limits on what the clinician can observe or infer about
the emotional aspects of motivation. For the most part, the clinician
evaluates motivation by focusing on patients' descriptions of their emotions, what they think about having them, and how they plan to control
or satisfy them.

There are three common situations in which the patient's motivations for suicide are likely to be assessed: when the patient has threatened suicide, has made a recent suicide attempt, or looks so depressed
or otherwise disturbed that the physician suspects suicidal motivation.
Dangerousness to others is assessed in analogous situations: when
the patient has threatened harm, has recently done harm to others, or
seems so emotionally disturbed that the physician suspects such harm
is possible.

Assessing the Motivation of the Patient Who Has Threatened Suicide

Communicating suicidal intentions to others is obviously not conducive to achieving the goal of suicide. The patient who tells others
about suicidal intent must, therefore, have motivations more complex
than a simple desire for self-destruction. There are many reasons why a
patient may threaten suicide, such as crying out for help, trying to gain
more attention, or wanting to hurt others. The first issue that the clinician must pursue is why the patient is making the threat. It is useful to
ask patients this question directly. They may not be able to answer it
directly, but replies such as "The pain is so bad I can't stand it anymore"
or "My life is horrible and there is no sign that it is getting better"
suggest that one major reason for making the threat is to receive help.
Patients rarely acknowledge the attention-seeking aspect of suicidal
threats. The clinician can learn about this type of motivation by asking
patients how they imagine others might respond to threats or to their

possible suicide. Questions such as "Who would be hurt the most if you actually did kill yourself?" or "Do your loved ones seem to care when you tell them how bad you feel?" are useful.

Sometimes, suicide threats are manipulative insofar as they are made to persuade others to behave in a certain way. Not infrequently, an individual abandoned by a lover threatens suicide in the hope that the threat will keep the relationship intact. Patients sometimes say to loved ones who want to leave them, "If I can't have you I would rather be dead: I will kill myself." Here, the implied threat of suicide may be clearly designed to elicit guilt, remorse, or fear in the person who wishes to leave. It is extremely important, however, for the clinician to realize that, although suicide threats are often made to gain attention or to manipulate others, the presence of such motivations does not necessarily diminish the risk of suicide. Patients have mixed motivations in threatening suicide. Though some of these may be attention-seeking or manipulative, this does not mean that other more "sincere" motivations of self-destruction are not present or that patients will not be pushed toward making a suicide attempt in an effort to prove the sincerity of their threat.

It is generally useful to ask patients about the depth of their suicidal intent by inquiring about what actual plans they have made for self-destruction and whether the means for implementing such plans are available. Patients who have made realistic plans to kill themselves are obviously at high risk. I have also found it useful to ask these patients, "What changes would have to take place in your life in order for you to feel that suicide is no longer a desirable option?" Most patients will then talk about possible changes in the way they feel or changes in their social or economic status that might make a significant difference. These are often issues that can be addressed in subsequent treatment. The patient who claims that nothing would make a difference poses a more serious problem and is generally at high risk of committing suicide because he is unwilling to consider other alternatives.

A related issue in dealing with threats is the importance of ascertaining whether the patient is actually communicating a threat. Some patients are very coy about suicidal intent. They may communicate a threat to one person but deny this intent when asked about it by others. Or they may be unresponsive when asked about suicidal intent by the clinician, refusing either to acknowledge or to deny it. Such patients may want more to gain attention or manipulate others than to receive help. There are also a group of patients who empathically insist that they wish they were dead. They may be very depressed but they may not be communicating a threat. Some of these patients may be thinking about suicide, but others are not motivated to hurt themselves, and although they may sincerely wish they were dead, they view *self*-destruction as morally repugnant.

The Patient Who Has Made a Suicide Attempt

In evaluating a patient who has made an unsuccessful suicide attempt, one of the clinician's major tasks is to assess the patient's motivation to persist in suicidal behavior. Often, suicide attempts appear to be
deliberately unsuccessful (for example, a patient may take ten aspirin or
make superficial cuts on a wrist), and there may be reason to believe that
self-destruction may not have been the patient's intent. This issue can
usually be clarified by asking the patient, "What were you hoping to
accomplish by this act?" or "Did you want to die?" It is also important
to determine how knowledgeable the patient is about what it takes to
kill oneself. Taking fifty milligrams of valium, for example, is not
necessarily a "gesture." The patient may have believed that this was a
lethal dose.

The question of why the patient made a suicide attempt should be
pursued with the same diligence used in pursuing the question of why
a patient made a suicidal threat. Knowledge about whether the patient
actually intended self-destruction may provide clues to the likelihood or
severity of a subsequent attempt. (Here, however, there are instances in
which the clinician can be misled by focusing too exclusively on the
patient's motivations. Some patients report that they had no intention of
killing themselves when they took an overdose or cut themselves and
that the act was motivated, rather, by a wish to influence others. These
patients may be quite sincere, but the clinician should always be aware
that anyone who makes a suicide attempt can underestimate the risks of
self-harm or overestimate the probabilities of being rescued.)

Making a suicide attempt generally has a profound effect on patients and their environments. Following an attempt, some patients develop an entirely new perspective on whether or not they want to die.
Environmental responses such as involuntary hospitalization and powerful emotional reactions toward patients on the part of their friends and
family will also influence future motivations. Some changes in the patient or in his or her environment may increase the likelihood of suicidal
behavior (for example, a minimal or angry reaction from loved ones, or
shame and greater depression because of having made the attempt), and
others may diminish it (for example, waking up after an overdose, realizing that the self-destructive act was unwise, and being very glad to
be alive, or a new and better understanding of one's problems by
one's family).

Much can be learned about the patient's postattempt motivations by
asking questions that assess the impact of the act itself. Questions such
as "Are you sorry or happy that you failed?" or "Are you embarrassed or
humiliated by what has happened?" or "Do you think having done this
will change your life in any way?" and particularly "How have others
responded to you since you made this attempt?" are useful.

158

CHAPTER SIX

Evaluating the Motivations of the Patient Who is Severely Depressed or Psychotic but Who Is Not Indicating Suicidal Intent

Often, patients, particularly those who are depressed or psychotic, appear to be suffering so greatly that, even though they voice no suicidal intent or vigorously deny it, the clinician still worries that they may be withholding or covering up self-destructive ideas. The kinds of questions that the clinicians ask in this situation were described in Chapter Three, and include "Do things seem hopeless?" and "How do you think this will all come out?" and "Have you felt so bad that you've had thoughts of hurting yourself in some way?" and "At your worst moments, do you ever think of hurting yourself?" Sometimes, these issues cannot be pursued too vigorously without destroying rapport with the patient. If the patient denies suicidal intent, and the clinician continues to ask questions such as "Are you suicidal?" the patient will feel that the doctor is not listening or simply does not believe him or her.

In these days of expanding malpractice litigation clinicians are sometimes advised to ask every depressed patient if he or she has motivations or plans for suicide. While asking these questions (and recording a negative answer) may help the clinician prevail in litigation if the patient should commit suicide, it is not good medical practice if it diminishes doctor–patient rapport. The clinician can usually gauge the explicitness of the questions needed to evaluate the individual patient's suicidal tendencies without having to ask questions that offend the patient.

Assessing the Motivations of the Patient Who Has Threatened Harm

When patients threaten harm to others, it is prudent to assume that they intend to carry out these threats. As in the case of suicidal threats, however, the clinician must also be concerned about other motivations for making threats, such as gaining power or attention or receiving help. It is easiest to begin an exploration of motivations by asking why the threat was made. Some patients insist that it was made in a momentary fit of anger and that all motivations to hurt the other person have disappeared. Other patients note that their threats were designed to impress other people or to change their behavior in some way but that they never really had any intention of carrying out the threats. Either of these kinds of responses may be genuine or dishonest. The clinician usually relies on other data to decide whether the patient still harbors an intent to commit harm.

When patients are direct in acknowledging current intent, the clinician needs to determine the depth of their motivations. Here, it is useful to examine the relationship between the patients and the persons or institutions they wish to harm. It is also useful to ask these patients whether they perceive violent motivations to be under the control of their own will. Persons who perceive themselves to be influenced by forces that they cannot control may not be fully deterred by fear of punishment.

Other questions that may help in assessing the intensity of the patient's motivation include "How carefully have you planned to commit this act?" and "Do you have the resources for doing it?" and "What do you think will happen if you actually do commit the act?" and "How will you feel afterward?" The latter two questions may be particularly important; where patients appear to be untroubled by the possible consequences of an aggressive act, such as punishment or feelings of guilt, motivations to commit harm are likely to be very strong.

Assessing the Motivations of the Patient Who Has Already Done Harm to Another Individual

When the patient has already committed a violent act, the clinician's major task is to determine the extent to which motivations to commit further acts of violence are still present. Some understanding of the patient's current motivation can be obtained by exploring the past violent act in detail. The clinician should focus on the environmental factors that preceded and followed the act as well as on how the patient felt before, during, and after the act. Exploring these issues gives some indication of the extent to which the patient experienced the act as controllable and may also uncover particular environmental contingencies that helped elicit the act, but that may or may not be present in future situations. An examination of the patient's thoughts and feelings in relation to the recent violent act will also give an indication of the depth of the patient's current motivations. Some violent acts are related to a specific type of emotional involvement with a specific person. The motivations that engender these acts may disappear once patients have been violent. There is a big difference between the patient who says, "After I hit him, I felt much better, and as far as I'm concerned I'm willing to forget about it," and the patient who says, "I know I hurt him a little, but I'm sorry I didn't kill him." It is also important to determine exactly who is at risk from the patient's violence. When violence appears to be directed at a specific person and at no one else, it may be possible to institute some simple remedial measures, such as ascertaining that the patient and the potential victim will not have contact with one another.

An act of violence, much like an act of suicide, is also likely to have profound consequences for the perpetrator. Sometimes, individuals who commit violent acts are hospitalized or arrested. They may be embarrassed, humiliated, or chastened by these events. They may feel extremely guilty about what they have done, or they may be angered that they have been apprehended. Violence also produces powerful and usually punitive responses from the patient's environment. The clinician needs to inquire how the patient has reacted to societal responses of arrest, imprisonment, or hospitalization. It is helpful to ask patients who have committed violent acts how they feel about what has happened to them subsequently. Another issue that is worth exploring is the capacity of violent patients to empathize with the plight of the individuals they have harmed. To the extent that patients compassionately understand what they may have done to others, they are more likely to experience some remorse, which may attenuate their violent motivations.

Assessing the Patient Who Has Neither Threatened nor Done Harm but Who Appears Capable of Violence

In dealing with patients with personality disorders, the clinician sometimes suspects that they are harboring motivations to do harm to others but are not talking about them. Some patients acknowledge these impulses if asked questions such as "Do you ever feel so angry that you feel you must do something to get even?" or "Do you spend much time thinking about trying to solve this problem by doing something illegal?" or "Do you ever feel that you might lose control of your anger?"

The evaluation of motivations for violence in psychotic patients is more difficult. This is true not only because these patients may have serious problems in communication. It is also likely that these patients experience violent motivations as sporadic and unpredictable, so that, at the time of the evaluation, they may be unaware of the existence of these motivations. In evaluating the possibility of violence by psychotic patients, the clinician must generally rely on knowledge of previous behavior and on nonverbal cues such as agitation, pacing about, threatening gestures, or signs of great fear. It is also useful to assess patients' delusional systems and to note carefully any beliefs that they have that others wish to harm them. Patients who truly believe that others wish them harm may strike out at those they mistakenly view as oppressors.

WHAT IS MEANT BY THE TERM *COGNITION* AND HOW IS OBSERVATION OF COGNITIVE PROCESSES RELEVANT TO PSYCHIATRIC EVALUATION?

Cognition is a general or generic term used to designate all processes involved in knowing. Most of the functions already discussed in this chapter are relevant to the process of knowing. The patient's emotional state certainly influences how he or she perceives, interprets, and uses knowledge. Disorders in the *form* of communication or thinking may be determined by pathological processes that prevent the patient from ordering and using knowledge. Disorders in the *content* of thinking are also aspects of cognitive impairment insofar as they are associated with false knowledge or inaccurate assessments of the environment. There are other psychological processes involved in the experience of knowing that have not yet been considered. These functions include perception, orientation, attention, memory, the ability to deal with abstractions, problem-solving ability, and judgment. The evaluator may also wish to observe the extent of the patient's current fund of knowledge, which gives a rough index of the intactness of the patient's cognitive functioning over time.

Patients cannot function unless they are able to accurately perceive, evaluate, and use information generated by environmental stimuli. The perceptual disorders that are most relevant to psychiatry involve gross misinterpretations of sensory input. Patients tend to report this type of deficiency spontaneously or to talk about these lapses after skillful inquiry.

Other cognitive abnormalities to be considered in this section, such as inability to sustain attention, disorientation, memory loss, or inability to deal with abstractions, are best viewed as signs rather than symptoms (although patients sometimes complain of problems in such functions as memory). These difficulties are either observed or detected by asking the patient more-or-less standardized questions, inquiries that can be viewed as tests. Evaluating this aspect of cognitive functioning puts the physician in the traditional medical role of testing the patient for signs of illness. This part of the study is sometimes called the *formal mental status examination*.

Cognitive functions that are formally tested are mediated by the cerebral cortex, and some cognitive deficits can be localized to specific cortical areas. Although this is not the only aspect of the mental status examination that tells about neurological deficits (certain motor abnormalities such as hyperactivity, hypoactivity, catatonia, echolalia, or echopraxia, for example, are also associated with frontal lobe dysfunction), it is the part of the mental status examination that tells us the most about it. Formal testing of cognitive functioning can be done with various degrees of precision and depth. Neuropsychologists have developed batteries of tests that are highly complex, that may take hours to administer, and that may precisely localize areas of cortical dysfunction. Psychiatrists generally limit themselves to relatively brief tests that take from five to twenty minutes. Such screening devices are usually adequate for picking up gross abnormalities. When more precise measurements of cognitive deficiency are required, or when the clinician suspects deficiencies but cannot detect them through routine types of questions, the patient is usually referred for neuropsychological testing.

WHAT ISSUES ARE IMPORTANT IN THE PSYCHIATRIC EVALUATION OF PERCEPTUAL IMPAIRMENTS?

The term *perception* refers to the processes by which an individual receives and interprets information from the environment. Environmental stimuli are mediated by the major sensory systems of the body: visual, auditory, olfactory, gustatory, tactile, kinesthetic, and visceral. The meaning of these stimuli is interpreted by the brain. The complexities of the perceptual processes are beyond the scope of this text, but it should be noted that perception is also influenced by other mental processes, such as the patient's emotional state.

In order to deal effectively with the environment, the patient must know it or perceive it accurately. Physical defects in sensory systems produce obvious perceptual handicaps. Psychiatric patients may have difficulty in accurately interpreting the environment specifically in the absence of any apparent physical abnormalities of the sensory systems. Patients may fail to respond to important stimuli, may misinterpret or distort stimuli, or may create false stimuli (that is, they may have perceptions in the absence of real or objectively observable stimuli).

At one time, psychiatrists dealt with a class of patients who were able to convince themselves and others that they had lost certain sensory functions, even when all sensory receptor systems were intact. These patients complained of varying degrees of blindness, deafness, or anesthesia but had no physical abnormality that would account for their deficits. They were described as having conversion reactions or conversion hysteria. Currently, psychiatrists in industrialized societies see few such patients. When patients with conversion reactions do appear, their perceptual defects are readily discerned from the nature of their complaints, from their attitudes toward their symptoms, and from the absence of any physical or neurological abnormalities.

Misperceptions of stimuli are more common; indeed, they are familiar with experiences. They occur in normal people who are fatigued or who are experiencing an intense emotional state such as anxiety. Most of us, when fatigued or anxious, have experienced real stimuli such as shadows or a heavy wind as something else (e.g., as a person or as a voice). These misperceptions of real stimuli are called *illusions*. They are especially common in children, who may experience them as frightening. Although illusions do not always suggest severe pathology, they are more common among seriously disturbed patients.

Perceptions can also be distorted. Sounds may appear to be louder or softer than their true intensity, or objects may be visualized as larger or smaller than their real size. Again, such distortions are usually associated with fatigue or intense emotional states such as anxiety, but the perception of objects as being larger (macropsia) or smaller (micropsia) than their true size may be associated with epileptic states.

The major disorder of perception that is of concern to psychiatrists is the phenomenon of hallucinations, that is, the occurrence of perceptions without discernible stimuli. In general, hallucinations, particularly if persistent, are an indication of a major psychiatric disorder. The only exceptions are the transitory hallucinations that occur in some people when waking (hypnopompic) or falling asleep (hypnogogic). Hallucinatory phenomena are intriguing to physicians because it is difficult to imagine what it would be like to experience regularly sensations that seem real in the absence of actual external stimuli. Indeed, psychiatrists have learned very little about how patients actually experience hallucinatory phenomena, perhaps because most patients who have such experiences are too disturbed to be accurate communicators. We do know that, for most patients, hallucinatory experiences are confusing and frightening.

The physician should examine the patient's hallucinatory experiences in as much depth as possible. Questions that should occur to the clinician immediately are "Do the patients know they are hallucinating?" and "Do the patients distinguish their perceptions as unrelated to real stimuli?" Patients who are experiencing delirium tremens (characterized by vivid visual hallucinations) may show a frightened response to their distorted perceptions; this response suggests that they have no idea that their perceptions are unreal. Similarly, patients who interrupt conversations with the examiner to talk or listen to an unseen person in the room are unlikely to appreciate the falseness of their perception. Patients who perceive the environment falsely and who are not aware that they are doing so are at a distinct social disadvantage. They are distracted from responding to real environmental stimuli and often convey to others a sense of being very disturbed.

If patients complain of or acknowledge hallucinatory phenomena, however, it is reasonable to assume that they have some awareness that their hallucinatory perceptions are different from their other perceptions. It is intriguing to investigate how this distinction is made. Some patients describe auditory hallucinations that consist of muffled voices, usually in the form of a few words or phrases whispered from inside their heads (these are called *incomplete auditory hallucinations*). It is relatively easy to understand how the patient can recognize this type of perception as unreal. When patients claim to hear voices that speak clearly from some location *other* than inside the head, it would appear that their discriminatory task is more difficult. Do patients hear the voices as unreal or different as a result of being unable to find their visual source, or do they distinguish them on the basis of their unusual pitch, intensity, or resonating quality? The clinician should try to inquire exactly where the voice seems to be coming from, the apparent sex of the speaker, and how the voice differs from ordinary voices. Sometimes, this inquiry yields much more than a better understanding of the patient. I once treated a schizophrenic patient who regularly heard the hallucinated voice of his mother. This distracted him at work until I was able to discover that there were no women in the room in which he worked. The patient learned not to respond to his hallucinations while at work—a small improvement, perhaps, but one that allowed him to retain his job.

The content of patients' hallucinations tells something about their problems. Patients in toxic states often have frightening visual hallucinations. On the other hand, the visual hallucination of a deceased love object or a romantic figure may be experienced as a pleasant experience; indeed, it can occur as a kind of wish fulfillment in bereaved or histrionic patients. Auditory hallucinations usually convey unpleasant messages, usually self-condemnatory. Sometimes, the hallucinated voice comments unfavorably on the patient's actions or repeats the patient's thoughts.

The clinician should also be alert to the existence of hallucinations that are neither visual nor auditory, but tactile, visceral, olfactory, or gustatory. The existence of these hallucinations is often revealed during the traditional medical history when various bodily systems are reviewed. In the process of the medical review of systems, the patient may make such statements as "Everything tastes strange," "I keep smelling burnt rubber," or "I feel as if there's some animal crawling around in my body." These perceptual disturbances should be carefully evaluated. Tactile, visual, olfactory, and gustatory hallucinations may occur in all types of psychotic conditions, but they should also alert the clinician to the possible existence of organic brain disease.

Several additional symptoms can be considered perceptual disturbances and are properly considered in this section of the mental status examination. Sometimes, patients complain of a disturbance in their sense of reality. They may complain that things seem unreal, unfamiliar, different, and strange. This symptom, called *derealization*, occurs with varying degrees of severity. It may be a transitory occurrence in nonpsychotic patients who are very anxious, but it is also commonly seen in the early stages of schizophrenia. A related symptom, called *depersonalization* is characterized by the patient's feeling that they are "not themselves." Not uncommonly, anxious patients complain of feeling different, and they may find that they observe themselves in a strange and detached way as they interact with others. This symptom occurs in many conditions and has little diagnostic significance. It does indicate, however, that the patient is experiencing a good deal of anxiety. As a rule, patients find the experience of depersonalization both interesting and frightening.

WHAT ARE SOME OF THE ISSUES INVOLVED IN
THE FORMAL TESTING OF COGNITIVE FUNCTIONS?

A great deal of information about the patient's cognitive functioning is obtained during the course of history taking; indeed, the history may yield most of what the clinician wishes to know. The physician who spends even a half hour with a verbally communicative patient generally learns a great deal about the patient's knowledge base, orientation, concentration, memory, and capacity for abstract thinking. For example, where patients meticulously state their problems, define the areas in which they are seeking help, and respond with precision to the physician's questions, it is easy for the clinician to infer that there is no impairment in concentration. The patient who remembers the dates and time sequences of recent and past events precisely can also be viewed as unlikely to have impairments in memory. Or the patient who comfortably uses metaphors and understands relationships and commonalities between events can generally be assumed to have good abstractive ability. Patients who describe various (realistic) options for dealing with their problems and the wisdom of following or not following them may be assumed to have good judgment.

Clinicians turn to testing when they wish to confirm their inferences about the patient's cognitive processes. In dealing with the majority of psychiatric patients, clinicians are wise not to trust their inferences fully and to test the various aspects of cognitive functioning formally. Usually, such testing merely confirms what the clinician already suspected. Quite frequently, however, the performance of patients on formal testing turns out to be different than would have been suspected from the observation of their capacities during interviews. Sometimes, the questions used in testing provide an additional bonus, insofar as the patient's answers may reveal aspects of the content of thought that were not apparent during history taking. This is especially likely when the patient is asked to interpret simple proverbs. Some patients may respond to this relatively ambiguous stimulus by discussing previously unrevealed delusional ideas.

Because, in the overwhelming majority of evaluations, the clinician does some kind of formal cognitive testing, almost every patient presents the physician with a challenge related to how and when such testing is to occur. One approach is to test cognitive functions as specific clues if cognitive impairments are elicited. If, for example, in describing the present illness, the patient is confused about dates, the clinician may wish to follow up on this symptom by interrupting the dialogue to ask questions about global orientation. Or if the patient is having obvious difficulty in remembering events, the clinician may empathically note that the patient is having difficulty with memory and may ask the patient to respond to some simple tests of memory. At first glance, this approach seems to have the advantage of relevancy and fluency. The examiner can test for cognitive deficiencies at a time when they are identified or suspected. There is no clumsy separation of conversational history taking and testing, and the physician does not have to search for a smooth means of introducing the subject of testing.

With all of the advantages of the above approach, it is not recommended here because of the subtle but powerful changes in the doctor-patient relationship that arise when the physician shifts to the role of formal tester. As long as the physician is taking a history in a conversational manner, the extent of his or her power over the patient is not emphasized. Most patients are willing to share intimate details of their difficulties with a wide variety of caring professionals and even with caring strangers. Asking the patient to answer test questions, however, changes the power balance between the participants in the interview. The physician becomes something more than a friendly listener. The patient is reminded that he or she is dealing with a physician whom society has granted the power to examine the thinking of patients, just as it has granted doctors the power to examine their bodies. (This part of the mental status examination can be conducted only if the patient consents to intrusions analogous to those involved in the physical examination.) Once any kind of testing begins, the relationship between doctor and patient becomes asymmetrical; in particular, the risk of the patient's confronting failure or embarrassment or discovering some major area of dysfunction is markedly increased.

If testing is separated from history taking, the physician has a different problem. A comfortable transition must be made to a more asymmetrical relationship in which the patient will very likely become more anxious. Typically, beginning clinicians have difficulty in making this transition and are either too abrupt (they may suddenly ask, "What day is it?") or too apologetic ("I just want to take a few minutes to ask you some silly, I mean, simple questions"). The approach recommended here is that a transitional statement be made by the physician in moving to testing, just as there is when the nonpsychiatric physician moves from history taking to physical examination. Some possible transitional phrases are "Before we end this interview, I do need to know a little bit more about some aspects of your thinking and understanding. I'd like to take a few minutes to ask you to answer some uncomplicated questions for me." Or the clinician may say, "I've learned a little bit about some of your thought processes from our conversation, but I'd like to take a few minutes to zero in on a few areas by asking you some questions that test some of your abilities."

Although I have discussed testing as a more-or-less formal function, it should be clear that asking the patient a few questions in the context of a psychiatric interview is hardly a very structured event. Nor is it every precise. The examiner's questions are not standardized. Nor are the patients prepared to use their maximum capacities as they would in a formal test situation. The testing of cognitive functions in the course of the mental status examination provides the physician with only a very rough idea of the patient's capacities. In my experience, most patients perform below their actual capacities on the cognitive aspects of the mental status examination. This is particularly likely to be true when such testing is done during the first interview. Furthermore, the patient who does poorly during the first interview is likely to do considerably better in the structured (and often more leisurely) context of formalized psychological testing.

Poor performance on cognitive testing cannot always be viewed as a sign of mental incapacity. The results can be affected by such factors as the patient's unusual anxiety during the psychiatric evaluation, the lack of standardization of the questions asked by psychiatrists, and inadequate responses arising from the patient's educational deficiencies or cultural differences. If deficiencies are found that do not fit in with the rest of the clinical picture presented by the patient, they must be investigated and reinvestigated by repeated testing, both within the interview context and with more sophisticated psychological tests.

HOW MUCH EFFORT SHOULD THE PSYCHIATRIST MAKE TO ASCERTAIN THE EXTENT OF THE PATIENT'S KNOWLEDGE BASE?

The extent of the patient's general information about the environment is often a critical factor in determining how successfully they interact with the environment. In most situations in life, knowledge is a key to power, and information about how the environment works and what it expects from the patient are critical to effective adaptation. Not all knowledge of the environment, of course, is directly translatable into greater adaptational potential, but as a general rule, those who seek and store information are in an advantageous position in dealing with most varieties of stress.

Traditionally, the assessment of an individual's fund of general information is based on the person's knowledge of current events, geography, or history. This knowledge can be tested by simply asking patients if they are aware of recent news events and, if they are, whether they can discuss them. Ordinarily, only knowledge of recent history is tested; patients are asked to name the current president and then to list, in the order of their service, as many previous presidents as they can. Sometimes, inquiries are made about the names of other political figures or other well-known historical figures. Geographical knowledge is tested by asking the patient to name state capitals, rivers, or mountains, or distances between various localities. These may be useful tests for people over forty. With the diminished attention to the teaching of geography in our schools for the last thirty-five years, the clinician often finds that even well-educated people under forty are abysmally ignorant of geography.

WHAT ARE THE CRITICAL ISSUES IN OBSERVING AND TESTING THE PATIENT'S ORIENTATION?

In order to deal effectively with the environment, the patient must have the capacity to be aware of its most basic physical elements. Patients who do not know precisely where they are or who they are interacting with have considerable difficulty in behaving adaptively. Patients who are unaware of the time of day and the date may be able to cope in an environment such as a hospital, where their needs are taken care of, but they are at a distinct disadvantage in a workplace environment. The patient's orientation to time, place, and person depends on a group of primitive cognitive functions (involving mental processes of both perception and memory) that are mediated by the frontal lobe. Patients who are disoriented in relation to time, place, or person usually have some type of organic brain disorder.

Disorientation can occur without organic brain disease; in particular, it may be present in situations where the patient lacks the motivation or the access to sensory cues that is required for orientation. Thus, patients who have been hospitalized for months may be unaware of the precise date, as they have no need of such an awareness. A stunned patient who wakes up in the hospital after an accident will initially be disoriented about place and person until provided with orienting information.

In the previous section, I stated that formal cognitive testing is best done in one block rather than interspersed throughout the interview; however, testing of orientation is sometimes an exception. Disoriented patients are likely to have difficulty providing accurate information throughout the interview. The sooner the interviewer knows about the existence of this deficit, the more accurately will he or she be able to fine-tune questions to the patient's capabilities and to gauge the reliability of the patient's answers. During history taking, if patients appear to be confused about recent time sequences, it is useful to inquire gently how long they have been in the hospital and the date of their admission. Patients who are unable to respond to these questions indicate sufficient lack of orientation so that it may not be necessary to ask, "What day is it today?" If patients complain of any kind of confusion or memory deficit, it is useful to ask them if they are having difficulty remembering dates, names, or locations. This approach can then lead to direct questions about orientation to time, place, and person.

When patients acknowledge disorientation or give obviously incorrect answers, they usually feel considerable anxiety or embarrassment. In conducting the remainder of the interview with such disoriented patients, the clinician must be especially empathic. It is useful to provide these patients with frequent orienting cues by periodically reminding them of the interviewer's name, why they are being interviewed, and the site of the interview.

WHAT ARE THE CRITICAL ISSUES IN OBSERVING AND TESTING THE PATIENT'S CONCENTRATION?

Concentration refers to the patient's ability to attend to environmental cues or to tasks. Any student knows that one's capacity to concentrate is related to many variables, including motivation, emotional state, and preoccupation with other stimuli. Thus, the student who is listening to a boring lecture, who is feeling anxious about his or her performance in that particular course, or who begins to stare at an attractive person in another part of the room will not concentrate very well on the subject material. On the other hand, after class, that same student may devote intense concentration to athletic events, playing video games, or reading an erotic novel. Severe deficits in the ability to concentrate may be related to frontal lobe dysfunction. In testing concentration, however, the examiner must first be concerned about what other psychological factors may be compromising the patient's willingness to focus on the task at hand.

Some patients complain of an inability to concentrate, and the clinician may be alerted to this possible cognitive deficiency from the beginning of the interview. Other patients may show deficits in concentration during the process of history taking; they may have difficulty in processing the examiner's questions and responding to them. In patients who give tangential or irrelevant responses which suggest poor concentration, however, a variety of psychological deficits other than impairment in concentration may account for their performance.

There are a number of traditional means of testing concentration, such as having the patient repeat a series of numbers in the order in which they were presented and then backward, subtract serial seven's, or spell various simple words backward. (These tests can also be viewed as tests of immediate recall.) Each of these tests should be given with very precise and simple instructions. When patients are presented with numbers that they are asked to repeat, the examiner should articulate the numbers slowly. It is appropriate to start out asking the patient to repeat numbers in the order in which the examiner presents them. When the examiner switches to asking the patient to repeat numbers in a reverse order, the new task should be clearly described. Many patients balk at subtracting serial seven's. Patients who profess to have difficulty with mathematics may be asked to do simpler mathematical tasks, such as subtracting serial three's, or to perform nonmathematical tasks of concentration, such as spelling words backward.

Sometimes, patients who seem quite attentive and responsive during the interview do quite poorly on formal tests of concentration. Indeed, the level of performance that patients achieve on formal testing of concentration cannot always be anticipated from their performance during the course of history taking. (Conversely, patients whose form of thinking during the interview suggests that they are not attending to the examiner's questions sometimes give quite precise answers on formal tests of concentration.) Unless patients perform substantially worse than has been anticipated from their previous educational achievements, the physician is wise not to jump to the conclusion that these patients are impaired. It is by no means certain that a patient who has difficulty repeating numbers backward or subtracting serial seven's has a true frontal lobe impairment; there are too many nonorganic causes of poor performance that need to be taken into consideration. Some textbooks claim that the normal person should be able to sequence five numbers backward and to subtract serial seven's without a mistake within ninety seconds; in fact, this is probably an unrealistic standard. In my experience, only about one out of twenty hospitalized patients I see comes up with this kind of performance.

WHAT ARE THE CRITICAL ISSUES IN OBSERVING AND TESTING THE PATIENT'S CAPACITY FOR ABSTRACT THINKING?

Abstract thoughts deal with ideas that are conceived apart from concrete realities, specific objects, or actual instances. Abstract thinking includes such psychological processes as forming concepts, categorizing information, generalizing from a single incident, applying procedural rules and general principles, and using metaphors. As a rule, abstract thinking is viewed as a "higher" cognitive function; accordingly, loss of the capacity to deal with abstractions is likely to be one of the first signs of organic brain disease.

Any demonstration of impaired abstractive ability usually requires some type of formal testing. However, the astute clinician can often suspect impairment in abstract thinking from the manner in which the patient goes about discussing historical data. Patients whose higher cognitive functions are impaired usually demonstrate a kind of thinking that it is referred to as *concrete*. They seem to be stimulus-bound and have difficulty in changing their responses or pulling their attention away from whatever happens to be their focus at a given moment. In the interview, they tend to become stuck on one track and unable to shift their frame of reference as the clinician seeks different levels of information. Other manifestations of loss of abstract capacity that may be noted during history taking are an inability to relate events to one another, to assess their importance and meaning, or to conceptualize aspects of one's interaction with the environment in the earlier phases of one's disturbance.

There are many sophisticated and standardized tests of the ability to deal with abstractions. Unfortunately, most of them are complicated and time-consuming. When time is limited, the clinician traditionally tests abstract thinking by asking patients to detect similarities and differences between various objects, to deal with simple mathematical thought problems, or to interpret proverbs. The test items in common use are generally borrowed from formal psychological tests. Over time, most physicians develop a series of favorite questions. The following are those I tend to use with most patients. I begin by asking the patient to describe commonalities or similarities between the following items: an orange and an apple, a bicycle and an airplane, a typewriter and a pencil, a fly and a tree, or a statute and a poem. If the patient has difficulty with any of these items, I switch to an easier item and go on to a different task. It is then useful to inquire about differences. The patient can be asked to describe the difference between a lie and a mistake, a midget and a small boy, or, if the patient is reasonably intelligent, between thrift and avarice or evolution and revolution. Because so many patients are terrified of responding to a mathematical thought problem, I generally pose only one very simple query: "If pencils are selling at two for ten cents, and if you have twenty-five cents and want to spend it all on pencils, how many pencils can you buy?" In my experience, only one out of five hospitalized patients answers this question correctly, and I am loathe to try any more difficult mathematical problem.

Some modern textbooks argue that the patient's responses to proverbs are rarely of any specific diagnostic value, and this may well be true. Responses to proverbs, however, are sometimes of great value in alerting the clinician to the possibility that the patient may be much sicker than was originally suspected. Moreover, they may also tell a great deal about the content of the patient's thinking. Not infrequently, a patient who shows no overt disturbance in the form or content of thought comes up with a totally inappropriate response when asked to interpret a proverb. Following up on a response that seems to make no sense often reveals the presence of delusional thinking. Patients who interpret proverbs in an eccentric or bizarre manner are also likely to go on talking about the associations generated by the proverb. Thus, they may reveal a great deal about the content of their preoccupations.

My practice is to regularly ask the patient to interpret two or three proverbs, usually beginning with a very simple one, such as "Don't cry over spilled milk" or "Every cloud has a silver lining." If the patient seems able to handle these (by giving a response that is not overly concrete), I move on to something slightly more difficult, such as "A bird in the hand is worth two in the bush" or "Don't put all your eggs in one basket." When patients appear to be doing well, I ask them to interpret the meaning of "A rolling stone gathers no moss." There are two possible meanings to this proverb (depending on whether moss is good or bad), and an intelligent, cognitively intact patient may come up with both of them. If proverbs are tactfully presented without stressing the patient, the interpretations of the proverbs often lead to an enjoyable form of interaction between physician and patient in which physician–patient rapport is enhanced and the physician's information is expanded.

WHAT ISSUES DOES THE CLINICIAN CONSIDER IN EVALUATING THE PATIENT'S JUDGMENT AND INSIGHT?

The mental function of judgment is one's capacity to evaluate information and to use this knowledge to plan for and deal with life situations. Judgment is frequently evaluated retrospectively on the basis of the patient's behavior. Patients who act in an inappropriate manner when they seem to have the capacity to do otherwise are often described as having poor judgment. The clinician must be wary, however, of assessing the capacity for judgment solely on the basis of the behavior. An individual may decide that stock market prices are soon going to drop precipitously but may be so preoccupied with other matters, so forgetful, or so self-destructive that he or she neglects to sell stock. This person has judged the situation correctly and the cognitive aspect of this judgment is intact. Although the ensuing behavior may be ineffective or maladaptive, it is not entirely a manifestation of defective judgment.

Tests of judgment in psychiatry focus on the patient's thinking about action and, specifically, on one's capacity for prospective planning. The traditional tests of judgment are "What would you do if you found a stamped, addressed, and sealed envelope on the street?" or "What would you do if you were in a crowded theater and were the first person there to discover a fire?" However, these queries detect only gross impairment in judgment. More practical information is obtained by focusing on how the patient goes about assessing and planning to deal with real-life problems. The existence of these problems becomes apparent during history taking. When patients describe problems dealing with other individuals or with their life situation, they can simply be asked, "How are you planning to deal with this situation?" or "What are your options?" or "What do you think will happen if you take no action?" The response to these questions generally gives some clues to how the patient has evaluated the situation and has planned to deal with it. With more sophisticated patients, the clinician may wish to inquire about the extent to which they can correctly identify the benefits, risks, and alternatives of various courses of action and can weigh these factors in planning what to do next.

WHAT ISSUES ARE INVOLVED IN
THE EVALUATION OF MEMORY?

Impairments in memory, even if minor, are generally distressing to patients. People are distinctly uncomfortable when they cannot remember the names of acquaintances. If they forget where they have parked their car, they may become extremely upset and may even experience panic. Subjective distress over memory impairment is not always communicated to the physician. Often, the patient who is so afflicted tries to hide this painful reality from family, friends, and the physician. Important exceptions to this observation are seriously depressed patients, who may exaggerate the degree of their memory impairment and may complain about the loss of capacities that they still retain.

Minor problems with memory occur in almost all psychiatric conditions characterized by anxious or depressed emotionality. The main concern of the physician, however, is with memory loss that is related to organic brain dysfunction. Organic memory loss is usually related to damage to the temporal lobes, but it may arise from damage to other parts of the cerebral cortex as well.

The functions of memory can be roughly categorized on a time scale, in terms of the remoteness of the events that are to be recalled. This classification is useful because loss of memory for more recent events is characteristically an early finding in organic disease. Memory is classified as immediate recall (the ability to remember something that has just happened), short-term recall (of events that happened only minutes earlier), recent recall (of events that occurred in the hours or weeks preceding the evaluation), and long-term, or remote recall (of events that happened years ago). Immediate recall is unlikely to be impaired in psychiatric patients. A loss of short-term or recent memory is much more common in anxious and depressed patients, as well as in those with organic brain disease. Long-term memory is unlikely to be impaired unless there is relatively advanced organic brain disease.

Immediate recall does not have to be formally tested; such a deficit would be manifest from the beginning of the interview in the patient's inability to respond to the examiner's questions. Short-term memory can be tested by asking patients to remember three or four items and by inquiring about their recollection of these items five minutes later. (In more formalized testing, standardized pairs of words can be taught to patients, and a few minutes later, they can be asked which words should be paired.) Recent memory is tested by asking patients about events in the previous twenty-four hours; either personal events, such as what they did or what they ate, or other environmental events, such as changes in the weather, of which they should be aware. Deficits in long-term memory may become apparent in the course of history taking, if the patient regularly seems confused about time sequences. Here, it may be useful to inquire about specific events in the patient's life, such as birth and marriage dates, job sequences, and the duration of past and present illnesses.

It is useful for the clinician to bear in mind that patients who do not have organic memory impairment may function quite poorly on tests of memory in the interview situation because of anxiety or lack of motivation to cooperate. When memory impairment is suspected on the basis of the mental status examination, it is generally useful to have the clinician's impressions of pathology substantiated by more formal psychological testing.

Some disorders of memory may not be aspects of the individual's current mental status but are likely to be observed as complaints in the course of history taking. These include an inability to recall events immediately preceding (retrograde amnesia) or immediately following (anterograde amnesia) a head injury. Other patients may experience and complain of a falsification of memory, noting that they feel that they have experienced an event before (*déjà vu*), or that they have had the rare experience of not recognizing a familiar situation (*jamais vu*). Traditionally, these symptoms are recorded in the mental status examination.

In assessing memory dysfunction, the experienced clinician learns to look for evidences that the patient is confabulating or fabricating information to compensate for knowledge that has not been stored or that cannot be recalled. Confabulation can be suspected when patients generalize in discussing an event of which they should have specific knowledge, or when they recount events in a manner that appears to be clearly inaccurate, bizarre, or unlikely.

WHAT ISSUES DOES THE CLINICIAN CONSIDER
IN EVALUATING THE PRESENCE OF APHASIA?

The term *aphasia* refers to a disturbance of language that is not caused by motoric irregularities of speech or articulation. It is manifested by linguistic dysfunction in the form of defective syntax, defective comprehension, or a loss of the capacity to choose words. Technically, it could be considered a disorder of thinking or of cognition, but because of its known neurological correlates, it is usually classified separately. For the most part, aphasia arises because of a brain lesion in the temporal cortex or in the posterior and inferior region of the frontal cortex of the dominant cerebral hemisphere. It is often associated with other neurological syndromes. When neurological symptoms are not manifest, aphasic patients may first be seen by the psychiatrist, who needs to be aware of any language dysfunction related to brain impairment.

Although the clinical picture of aphasia is complex and variable, aphasic disorders are generally classified into two broad categories. In Broca's aphasia or frontal aphasia, verbal expression is severely impaired, but the patient can comprehend both spoken and written language. In Wernicke's aphasia, the speech is fluent and well articulated but the patient has difficulty comprehending what is heard and, sometimes, what is seen. Patients with Broca's aphasia tend to speak slowly and laboriously, using mainly nouns and verbs. This type of aphasia is classically tested for by asking the patient to repeat phrases or sentences, such as "Methodist Episcopal" or "no if's, and's, or but's." Patients with such an expressive aphasia have great difficulty in repeating these phrases fluently. On the other hand, they should have no difficulty naming or recognizing objects. They can generally name objects that the examiner points to and can almost always point to objects such as their own body parts, clothing, or office paraphernalia if the examiner asks them to.

In Wernicke's aphasia, the patient is likely to be more seriously disabled, and the diagnostic problem for the psychiatrist is usually more complex. These patients may speak fluently, but there is a distortion in the relatedness of their ideas. Because they have an incapacity to comprehend what they hear and often what they see, their language is likely to be characterized by jargon, disconnected ideas, and the use of neologisms and word approximations. When asked to repeat a phrase such as "Methodist Episcopal," they may not respond, as they may not comprehend the request. Individuals with Wernicke's aphasia can be distinguished from schizophrenic patients on the basis of history and testing. Language disorders related to cerebral impairment generally have a rapid onset, as opposed to an insidious development in patients with schizophrenia. Most schizophrenic patients are also able to respond to simple verbal directions, such as pointing out items of clothing, body parts, or office paraphernalia, whereas patients with Wernicke's aphasia cannot do so.

WHAT ASPECTS OF PARIETAL LOBE FUNCTIONING CAN BE TESTED IN THE COURSE OF THE MENTAL STATUS EXAMINATION?

The dominant parietal lobe generally influences verbal and symbolic abilities, and the nondominant parietal lobe influences nonverbal motor-perceptual abilities. Impairment in parietal lobe functioning is more likely to present as a neurological than as a psychiatric problem, but sometimes, the impairment—or the patient's response to the impairment—is quite similar to the symptomatology seen in certain psychiatric syndromes. Psychiatrists do not ordinarily test parietal lobe functioning and tend to leave this task to neuropsychologists and neurologists; there are, however, certain motor and cognitive impairments that are relatively easily tested during the course of the mental status examination. The psychiatric clinician should be aware of these and should be able to do at least a general screening for parietal dysfunction.

Parietal lobe dysfunction may be manifested by the patient's inability to perform everyday motor behaviors, even though there is no sensory loss or muscular incapacity. This impairment is called an *apraxia* and can be tested for by asking the patient to perform simple tasks. When asked to perform an action from memory, patients with lesions in the dominant parietal lobe may be unable to do so without props (ideomotor apraxia). If asked to demonstrate the use of a key or a hammer with each hand, they may be unable to comply. Patients with a kinesthetic apraxia may be unable to copy various movements that the examiner models and asks the patient to repeat. Patients with nondominant parietal lobe lesions may have difficulty copying simple figures, such as a cross or a square, without removing their pencil from the paper.

Patients with dominant parietal lobe lesions may also have spatial categorization problems. They may exhibit right–left disorientation. This can be tested for by asking patients to touch one part of their body to a contralateral part (for example, "Touch your right hand to your left toe"). Another symptom of dominant parietal lobe dysfunction is an inability to name one's own fingers correctly (finger agnosia).

Other symptoms associated with dominant parietal lobe disorders include difficulty in performing mathematical calculations (dyscalculia), difficulty in writing (dysgraphia), or difficulty in reading (dyslexia). These functions can be tested by asking patients to do very simple calculations, by asking them to write some sentences (preferably in script), and by asking them to read aloud.

Finally, the clinician should be aware that lesions of the nondominant parietal lobe may be associated with a diminished capacity to recognize certain aspects of the environment or of one's own body (usually on the left side). There may be a denial of illness, a denial of the existence of body parts, and an uncertain recognition of familiar people. Such complaints are very similar to those seen among highly disturbed psychiatric patients. The so-called Capgras syndrome (in which the patient insists that familiar people are actually imposters or doubles) can be produced by a parietal lobe lesion.

FOR FURTHER READING

Alexander, M. P. Clinical determination of mental competence. *Archives of Neurology*, 45:23, 1988.

Detre, T. P., and Jarecki, H. G. *Modern psychiatric treatment*. Lippincott, Philadelphia, 1971.

Havens, L. L. The need for tests of normal functioning in the psychiatric interview. *American Journal of Psychiatry*, 141:1208–1211, 1984.

Leon, R. L., Bowden, C. L., and Fayber, R. A. The psychiatric interview, history and mental status examination. In *Comprehensive textbook of psychiatry*, Vol. 5, H. I. Kaplan and B. J. Sadock (Eds.). Williams & Wilkins, Baltimore, 1989.

Lezak, M. D. *Neuropsychological assessment* (3rd ed.). Oxford University Press, New York, 1974.

MacKinnon, R. A., and Yudofsky, S. *The psychiatric evaluation in clinical practice*. Lippincott, Baltimore, 1986.

Menninger, K. A., Mayman, M., and Pruyser, P. W. *A manual for psychiatric case study* (2nd ed.). Grune & Stratton, New York, 1962.

Pruyser, P. W. *The psychological examination: A guide for clinicians*. International Universities Press, New York, 1979.

Scheiber, S. C. Psychiatric interviews, psychiatric history and the mental status examination." In *Textbook of psychiatry*, J. A. Talbott, R. E. Hales, and S. C. Yudofsky (Eds.). American Psychiatric Press, Washington, D.C., 1988.

Sims, A. *Symptoms in the mind: An introduction to descriptive psychopathology*. Baillier-Tindall, London, 1988.

Stubb, R. L., and Black, F. W. *The mental status examination in neurology*. F. A. Davis, Philadelphia, 1977.

Taylor, M. A. *The neuropsychiatric mental status examination*. S. P. Medical and Scientific Books, New York, 1981.

Taylor, M. A., Sierles, F., and Abrams, R. The neuropsychiatric evaluation. In *American Psychiatric Association Annual Review*, Vol. 4, pp. 109–141, R. F. Hales and A. J. Francis (Eds.). American Psychiatric Press, Washington, D.C., 1985.

Wells, C. E. Pseudodementia. *American Journal of Psychiatry*, 136:895, 1979.

CHAPTER SEVEN

Additional Procedures and Tests in the Diagnostic Process, Laboratory Testing, Electroencephalogram, Imaging, and Psychological Testing

There are a number of procedures and tests that the psychiatric clinician can use to facilitate the assessment process. Although these procedures and tests are usually referred to as *diagnostic*, they do not always clarify diagnostic issues; indeed, in many instances, they are better thought of as tests of pathogenicity or etiology.

Currently, there is a wide gap between the clinical and the research yields that are obtained by means of laboratory and other testing. Many of the testing procedures that are currently available have limited *clinical* usefulness but are very promising *research* instruments. The focus in this chapter is to review briefly those procedures and tests that are generally agreed to have clinical usefulness. Accordingly, such tests as the dexamethazone suppression test (DST) or the thyroid-releasing hormone test (TRH), which are very important research instruments, will not be discussed here. Although some believe that these tests do have clinical usefulness, the preponderance of current opinion is that they do not offer sufficiently precise information to regularly guide the clinician in prescribing treatment.

In determining whether and when to order a specific test, the clinician considers two major issues. First, what guides do the history, the mental status examination, and the physical examination offer to the possible causes of the patient's illness that must be further investigated if rational treatment is to be provided? Any psychiatric finding that suggests organic impairment, for example, must be fully investigated for a determination of the precise nature of the processes involved. Second, the physician should consider whether the possible yield or gain from testing will be significant enough to outweigh the possible disadvantages to the patient. Obviously, any knowledge gained by testing is useful; on the other hand, testing has both an economic and a personal cost to the patient. The latter includes time demands, potential embarrassment, discomfort, fear, (particularly for procedures such as CAT), and possible adverse side effects.

In these days of economic restraints in medical practice, there is pressure on the physician to be conservative when ordering tests. In terms of the quality of patient care, however, this is one area in which conservatism may be unwise. The benefits of testing ordinarily far outweigh its risks, and it is only when this is not the case that testing should be limited. If the patient's condition is deteriorating or not improving, the physician is always wise to err on the side of over- rather than undertesting.

WHEN SHOULD THE CLINICIAN TEST FOR ORGANICITY?

Many symptoms of mental illness are caused by measurable anatomical and physiological variations. If these variations can be precisely defined, the clinician may be able to treat them and to provide the patient with considerable relief. Even if the anatomical and physiological variations cannot be effectively treated, the clinician can often surmise how these deficiencies will limit the patient's present and future capacities. For example, if a patient has sustained a serious head injury and has lost significant cognitive skills, it is extremely useful for the clinician to know how the patient has been functionally compromised, and what the likelihood is that the impairment is treatable. This information enables the physician to advise patients to assume only those tasks that are within their capacities and to advise family members about what to expect of the patients. Such advise giving is an extremely important, if unspectacular, part of psychiatric treatment.

In thinking about the issue of organic causation in psychiatry, the clinician must recognize that any disorder or behavior or experience can have an organic cause. Some symptom clusters, however, are very likely to be associated with detectable organicity, whereas others are not. Knowledge of organic causation may determine the choice of treatment, or it may tell a great deal about the patient's prognosis. Vigorous testing for organicity is always indicated when there is a high probability that a given symptom cluster has a known organic factor in its pathogenesis.

Certain behavioral or experiential syndromes are very likely to be caused by a detectable organic impairment. The most common are those associated with the syndrome of delirium, in which the patient experiences a diminished capacity both to sustain attention to environmental stimuli and to perceive them accurately. The patient's incapacities are likely to be manifested by a variety of symptoms, some of which may change very quickly. Delirious patients may be agitated or lethargic, inattentive or hypervigilant. They may be disoriented, have memory impairments, speak incoherently, and complain of hallucinations. Diagnosing the cause of delirium is critical because the organic condition may be at once life-threatening and treatable. Delirium is commonly seen on medical wards, where it is most likely to be caused by hypoxia, hypoglycemia, excessive use of sedative medications, or drug overdose. In the emergency room, delirium is usually associated with drug intoxication or withdrawal.

The syndrome of dementia is also caused by detectable organic dysfunction. In dementia, there is no clouding of consciousness, but memory impairment is present along with a diminished capacity for abstract thinking and, usually, impaired judgment. Patients with dementia may also become depressed in response to their loss of cognitive capacity. Dementia can be caused by almost any pathological process that influences the brain, including trauma, infection, toxicity, tumors, and disturbed nutrition, as well as endocrine, vascular, autoimmune, metabolic, and degenerative diseases. The clinician should also be aware that symptoms similar to those of dementia may be evidenced by severely depressed patients who do not have any of the above-listed pathologies. These patients (who are described as having pseudomentia) regain their cognitive capacities when their depression is successfully treated. They are generally distinguished from the demented group by having a history of psychiatric difficulty, by an acute rather than an insidious onset of cognitive impairment, by little effort to conceal (and even a tendency to exaggerate) their symptoms, and by a loss of remote as well as recent memory.

Even though some of the processes that cause dementia are irreversible, it is always important to determine the pathogenesis of this condition. A knowledge of the causes of dementia helps the clinician to deal with other aspects of that disease and to initiate preventive measures that may keep the patient from becoming worse. It also helps the physician to advise patients and their families properly about prognosis.

The likelihood that the psychotic symptomatology associated with schizophrenia or bipolar illness (patients with these disorders rarely show clouding of consciousness or loss of memory) has a detectable organic etiology is less than can be anticipated if the presenting symptoms are those of delirium or dementia. Any of the organic brain syndromes, however, including dementia, may initially present with symptoms of psychosis, such as delusions, hallucinations, flattened affect, or deviations in the form of thought, rather than with disruptions of intellect. It is therefore very important to exclude organic etiology when the symptoms appear to be those of the so-called functional psychoses. When a psychotic process is acute, the clinician should always suspect a disruption in brain functioning on a metabolic or toxic basis. Special attention should be paid to the possibility of drug intoxication involving stimulants or hallucinogens.

The symptoms associated with anxiety and the nonmanic mood disorders are least likely to have a detectable organic pathogenesis. When these are the presenting conditions, the degree of urgency in ruling out organicity is ordinarily less than in the case of syndromes such as delirium, dementia, or psychosis. Nonetheless, the clinician must be aware of the large number of organic conditions that can cause anxiety or depression. Endocrinopathies, particularly those involving the thyroid or the adrenal cortex, are relatively common etiological factors. Less likely possibilities are hypo- and hyperparathyroidism, pheochromocytoma, or hypoglycemia. Patients with neurological, metabolic, and chronic systemic disorders, as well as neoplasms, may initially present with depressive symptomatology.

Although the psychiatrist must be extremely conscientious in ruling out organicity, he or she must also be aware that organic causation will *not* be found in most psychiatric patients. Even when organic changes are found to be associated with symptoms of psychosis, anxiety, or depression, it cannot always be said that these changes are etiological. (Organic findings can be incidental as well as etiological, or they may develop, in part, in response to the mental disorder.) It is also true that psychiatric patients sometimes exaggerate or develop symptoms that mimic those of the more common brain diseases or of nonpsychiatric medical disorders. As noted previously, depressed patients may appear to be demented when they are not (pseudodementia). Anxious patients often worry about their health and develop physical symptoms that are unrelated to a detectable organic disorder. Patients with somatoform or factitious disorders may present with symptoms highly suggestive of medical disorders, but they will have no detectable structural or physiological pathology.

In dealing with the majority of psychiatric patients, the clinician's task is one of doing enough investigation of organic etiology to be able to assure the patient that it is not detectable. Considerable skill is then required in presenting this information to the patient. There are many psychiatric patients who respond to the physician's message "You are in good physical health" with concerns that this means that their symptoms are "all in their head" and with the fear that they will be blamed for their symptoms and viewed by others (and themselves) as willfully creating them. Anxious and depressed patients may actually wish that some minor organic etiology of their condition could be found, so that they did not have to feel responsible for their symptoms. Psychiatric patients who are suffering, but who happen to be in good physical health, should never be told that they are free of illness. Rather, a message like the following is preferred:

> It appears at this time that we can detect no organic cause for your symptoms. This is really good news. It means we have ruled out a lot of serious possibilities. Still, I know you are suffering and need treatment. You do have an illness, which is likely to respond either to medicine or to some other form of psychiatric treatment. You are not responsible for your suffering. You do, however, have choices in what to do about it, and you are responsible for cooperating in the treatment I will prescribe.

Patients often do inquire about whether they are responsible for their symptoms. This may be as useful a place as any to consider how the clinician should respond to such questions. The question of how doctors, patients, and their families attribute responsibility for symptoms is very complex, yet the issue has ramifications with which the physician must deal on a daily basis. When patients ask, "Have I caused my illness?" or "Is it all in my head?" or when relatives or hospital staff ask, "Can he control this behavior?" or "Should we try to prevent him from sitting in his room all day?" the physician must come up with answers. One simple rule that I have found useful is to tell patients that they should never blame themselves for their feelings. They cannot will themselves to feel better. I also tell them that they have at least a little control over their thinking, and that it may be helpful for them to try to think more positively and rationally. Most important, I remind them that they almost always have some control over their behavior. In this approach, a typical depressed patient on an inpatient unit would be told that one is not responsible for feeling anxious or depressed. The patient would also be educated, however, about how thoughts can be partially controlled so as not to escalate symptoms. At the same time, the patient would be reminded that one can almost always exert some control over behavior and would be held responsible for actions such as eating, going to ward activities, talking to therapists, and taking medication.

WHAT TESTS SHOULD THE PHYSICIAN USE TO INVESTIGATE ORGANICITY?

The precise test(s) that the clinician uses to investigate organicity will, of course, vary with the nature of the psychiatric and physical findings. However, there are some general rules that the clinician can follow in dealing with various clinical presentations.

Because delirium is an acute, medical emergency, it should be investigated through a screening profile that includes serum glucose, electrolytes, enzymes, blood urea nitrogen, serum alcohol, a complete blood count, and a urine drug screen. Arterial blood-gas analysis, lumbar puncture, or cranial CT may also be ordered as indicated. Electroencephalography may be useful if the patient's condition is not very serious, and if he or she is cooperative. The clinician should also be concerned about the possibility that psychiatric patients may be receiving toxic doses of psychotropic medications and may wish to test for tricyclic levels when anticholinergic symptoms are prominent.

The laboratory evaluation of dementia need not be as hurried as that for delirium, as dementia is a more chronic and not an acutely life-threatening condition. Dementia patients, however, are quite susceptible to delirium, and the clinician should be quick to suspect delirium if these patients show any unusual change in their capacity to sustain attention. Although the establishment of some causes of dementia does not currently provide guidelines to remedial treatment (Alzheimer's disease is the most depressing example), there are some dementias that are treatable. Accordingly, the clinician should direct laboratory testing toward finding a treatable cause. The *routine* screening should include electrolytes, liver and renal function tests, a twelve-parameter metabolic screen, a complete blood count (CBC) with differential, thyroid function tests, serology for syphilis, a chest X ray, electrocardiography (EKG), and CT. Other procedures may be used as well, depending on what diagnostic cues are obtained from the history and the physical exam. Such studies include blood and urine screens for alcohol, drugs, and heavy metals: an HIV antibody test, tests for arterial blood gases, and serum and urine copper, and electroencephalography (EEG). When dementia is suspected, CT of the head is always indicated; however, the clinician must appreciate the limitations of this procedure. Severely demented Alzheimer's patients may have normal CT scans, whereas elderly patients without dementia may show considerable cerebral atrophy.

When patients display symptoms of psychosis without the perceptual and cognitive abnormalities seen in delirium and dementia, the approach to laboratory testing is more problematic and depends on the acuteness of the disorder. If a patient presents with symptoms of psychosis for the first time (even if the patient's sensorium is clear), the physician should still rule out the possibility of metabolic or toxic disorder. The tests used here are similar to those used in determining the causes of delirium, with a special emphasis on ruling out drug intoxication. In younger patients, the chance of finding an organic disorder during the initial presentation of psychosis is remote. Nonetheless, it is imperative that the search be made, not only to give a more definitive diagnosis, but also to allow the patient to be given an explanation of what has happened. (A psychotic experience is much less terrifying if it can be explained by some controllable event, such as drug intoxication.)

In patients with more chronic psychosis, the search for organicity is generally less urgent and includes the kinds of tests used in the evaluation of dementia.

The majority of psychiatric patients seek help for anxiety or depression. Even if the patient's primary problem is a personality disorder, it is usually the experience of anxiety or depression that initiates the search for help. Such experiences can also be directly associated with an organic disorder that involves the central nervous system.

Although there is a temptation to assume an absence of organicity in patients who present with symptoms of anxiety or depression, in each case the clinician should always do a medical work-up including a medical history and a physical examination. The findings may suggest specific areas of pathology to be evaluated. Even if the medical history and examination do not suggest organic pathology, there are certain routine laboratory tests that should be considered. The patient who presents with anxiety or depression for the first time, or who has recurrent symptoms but has not been medically evaluated for over a year, should receive a CBC with differential; a biochemical profile including electrolytes, glucose, hepatic and renal functions, calcium and phosphate levels; a urinalysis; and a thyroid function test. Depending on the nature of the symptomatology (and other information obtained in the medical history and the physical examination), further procedures, including a chest X ray, an EKG, an EEG, folate and B-12 tests, a test for syphilis, and drug screening, should be considered.

In patients who present with symptoms of depression, thyroid function testing is especially important. Hypothyroidism can be a sufficient and necessary cause of depression. Knowledge of this etiology significantly enhances the prospects for treatment. The tests most commonly used to screen for hyperthyroidism are measurements of serum, T-3, and T-4. More accurate tests of thyroid functioning can be obtained by combining several tests of hypothalamic-pituitary-thyroid gland functions. Although there is controversy about whether more sophisticated measurements of thyroid functioning (such as the TRH test) are needed with every depressed patient, there is general agreement that some measure of thyroid function is desirable.

WHAT ARE THE MAJOR INDICATIONS FOR THE USE OF COMPUTERIZED TOMOGRAPHY AND THE ELECTROENCEPHALOGRAM IN PSYCHIATRY?

Computerized tomography (CT) is a radiological technique that allows the visualization of anatomical disturbances in the brain. These include lesions larger than 1.5 centimeters, ventricular displacement or change in size, and abnormal brain tissue. Magnetic resonance imagery (MRI) provides an even more precisely defined image of brain tissue but is generally more expensive and time-consuming than CT. Some general indications for CT in psychiatry are:

1. The presence of confusion associated with delirium.
2. Dementia.
3. Movement disorders.
4. Anorexia.
5. Prolonged catatonia.
6. The first episode of an affective disorder in a patient over fifty.

The CT scan requires a reasonably cooperative patient who can tolerate the stress of lying in a small, enclosed space for at least fifteen minutes.

The electroencephalogram is an important screening test for organicity and may reveal abnormalities that are not of sufficient anatomical magnitude to be apparent on CT. This test is indicated in delirium, in dementia, in psychosis that appears for the first time, and in any situation in which behavioral changes might be explained as a form of a seizure disorder. The latter category would include impulse disorders and pathological responses to alcohol ingestion.

WHAT PSYCHOLOGICAL TESTS ARE MOST USEFUL IN PSYCHIATRIC EVALUATION?

Traditionally, psychological tests have been used by psychiatrists to confirm diagnostic impressions and to obtain additional information about the patient's psychological functions that may be relevant to treatment. They generally provide information about intelligence, personality variables, or neuropsychological impairment. Sometimes, a single test such as the Wechsler Adult Intelligence Scale—Revised (WAIS-R) provides information in all of these areas.

The use of these tests in psychiatry is often determined by both the setting in which the patient is evaluated and treated and the attitudes and orientation of the clinician. Hospitalized patients, who generally have more serious disorders, regularly receive more testing than do outpatients. The nature of the hospital also makes a difference. Private hospitals generally do more intensive testing, and long-term hospitals put more emphasis on the use of projective tests of personality, such as the Rorschach and the Thematic Apperception Test (TAT). Projective tests are especially useful in providing psychodynamic insights.

Hospitals that provide shorter term treatment and nonpsychiatric medical units may rely on nonprojective personality tests such as the MMPI, which can be administered and scored with little use of the physician's time. Evaluations done for legal purposes are likely to include a great deal of psychological testing because the use of these tests is viewed as evidence of thoroughness in the evaluative approach, and because judicial agencies (rightly or wrongly) tend to view tests as having more validity than clinical impressions.

With the exception of neuropsychological testing, most psychiatric evaluation and treatment can be done reasonably well without the use of psychological testing. In most situations, psychological testing is best viewed as an adjunct source of information. Clinicians who are not certain of their diagnoses or who need to know more about the cognitive style or personality of their patients may wish to obtain additional information through the use of tests such as the Rorschach, the TAT, or the MMPI. Many clinicians who adhere to a psychodynamic approach may routinely request projective personality tests. Certainly, clinicians who know that their reports will be scrutinized by legal agencies may be motivated to use such tests regularly. In ordinary practice, however, clinicians use testing in a more discriminatory fashion, primarily when they feel uncertain about a diagnosis or about the most expeditious treatment approach.

Neuropsychological testing is an exception. Many brain lesions elicit behavioral and experiential changes long before neurological impairments are obvious. Neuropsychological tests, which measure functional brain capacities, may be able to uncover cerebral incapacities that cannot be detected by laboratory testing, CT, or the EEG. They provide more precise measurements of memory, intelligence, judgment, perception, motor capacity, sensory capacity, language use, and mental flexibility than can be obtained in a routine mental status examination. Tests such as the WAIS-R, the Bender Visual-Motor Gestalt, the Vineland Social Maturity Scale, the Purdue Pegboard Test, the Language Aphasia Battery, and test batteries such as the Halstead-Reitan or the Luria-Nebraska Neuropsychological Examination, may be especially useful in detecting early brain dysfunction.

Generally, neuropsychological testing has both diagnostic and therapeutic implications. The more sophisticated test batteries can establish the existence of cognitive and behavioral deficits. Sometimes, they help in the localization of lesions and provide data about their severity and magnitude. Equally important from a therapeutic standpoint, these tests can provide information about the remaining strengths and weaknesses of organically impaired patients and may offer clues to the patient's ability to function at work or at home. This information has obvious implications for rehabilitation strategies.

Although neuropsychological testing is not used as frequently as medical procedures such as imagery or EEG techniques (perhaps because insuring agencies, including Medicare, are reluctant to pay for it), my view is that it is an essential tool in the diagnosis and treatment of any patient suspected of having an organic brain injury. Its therapeutic aspects are especially important because it provides the clinician with relatively precise data about what patients can be expected to accomplish, and what they may be unable to do. Again, such information is highly useful to members of the patient's family, who must understand his or her limitations while helping him or her to make the best use of all remaining capacities.

FOR FURTHER READING

Anastasi, A. *Psychological testing* (5th ed.). Macmillan, New York, 1982.

Bigler, E. D. *Diagnostic clinical neuropsychology.* University of Texas Press, Austin, 1984.

Boll, T. J. The Halstead-Reitan Neuropsychology Battery. In *Handbook of clinical neuropsychology*, S. B. Filskov and T. J. Boll (Eds.). Wiley, New York, 1987.

Clarkin, J. F., and Hurt, S. W. Psychological assessment: Tests and rating scales. In *American Psychiatric Association textbook of psychiatry.* American Psychiatric Press, Washington, D.C., 1988.

Crosse, J. B., Olin, C. M., and Morihisa, J. M. Brain imaging and lab testing in neuropsychiatry. In *A textbook of neuropsychiatry.* American Psychiatric Press, Washington, D.C., 1987.

Cummings, J. L., and Bensdon, D. F. *Dementia: A clinical approach.* Butterworth, Boston, 1983.

Dubovsky, S. L. *Concise guide to clinical psychiatry*, Chapter 5. American Psychiatric Press, Washington, D.C., 1988.

Franzen, M. D., and Lovell, M. R. Neuropsychological assessment. In *Textbook of neuropsychiatry.* American Psychiatric Press, Washington, D.C., 1987.

Golden, C. J. *Clinical interpretation of objective psychological tests.* Grune & Stratton, New York, 1979.

Groth-Marnot, G. *Handbook of psychological assessments.* Van Nostrand & Reinhold, New York, 1984.

Hall, R. C. W., and Beresford, T. P. *Handbook of psychiatric diagnostic procedures, Vols. 1, 2.* Spectrum Publications, Jamaica, N.Y., 1984.

Hall, R. C., Beresford, T. P., and Gardner, B. R. The medical care of psychiatric patients. *Hospital and Community Psychiatry, 33:25*, 1982.

Halsted, J. A., and Halsted, C. H. *The laboratory in clinical medicine: Interpretations and applications* (2nd ed.). W. B. Saunders, Philadelphia, 1981.

MacKinnon, R. A., and Yudofsky, S. C. *The psychiatric evaluation in clinical practice*, Chapters 3, 5. Lippincott, Philadelphia, 1986.

Nasrallah, H. A., and Koffman, J. A. Computerized tomography in psychiatry. *Psychiatric Annals, 4:2, 39*, 1985.

Rainey, J. M., and Nesse, R. M. Psychobiology of anxiety and anxiety disorders. *Psychiatric Clinics of North America, 8:133*, 1985.

Reitan, R. M., and Davison, L. A. *Clinical neuropsychology: Current status and applications.* Winston Press, Washington, D.C., 1974.

Rosse, R. B. Laboratory and other diagnostic tests in psychiatry. In *American Psychiatric Association textbook of psychiatry*. American Psychiatric Press, Washington, D.C., 1988.

Sternberg, D. E. Biological tests in psychiatry. *Psychiatric Clinics of North America, 7*:639, 1984.

Weinberger, D. R. Brain disease and psychiatric illness: When should a psychiatrist order a CAT scan? *American Journal of Psychiatry, 14*:1521, 1984.

Wise, M. G., and Rundell, J. R. *Concise guide to consultation psychiatry*, Chapter 3. American Psychiatric Press, Washington, D.C., 1988.

CHAPTER EIGHT

Evaluation of Capacities in Psychiatry

In Chapter One, I noted that one major way in which a psychiatric evaluation differs from evaluations in other medical specialties is the extent to which it is focused on an assessment of the patient's capacities. I also noted the failure of psychiatric educators to develop models for teaching students how to evaluate capacities. In many ways, that failure is understandable. The evaluation of capacities requires a great deal of conceptualization and speculation about the interaction of many biological, psychological, and social variables. Often, the task involves making predictions on the basis of insufficient data. Sometimes, the evaluation may even take on a moral dimension.

In this chapter, I suggest a conceptual framework that can be used in evaluating capacities. It should be clear that no definitive model for evaluating capacities actually exists, and that this chapter will not remedy that lack. The most that I hope to accomplish is to list the factors that the student should consider in making these evaluations, and to suggest ways of thinking about them in an organized manner. This approach is taken on the basis of a firm belief that learning and skill development proceed more efficiently if the student systematically conceptualizes clinical decisions, instead of relying exclusively on the uncertain reed of clinical intuition.

WHAT CAPACITIES ARE EVALUATED IN PSYCHIATRY?

One convenient way of classifying the capacities of concern to psychiatrists is as past (retrospective), present (contemporaneous), or future (prospective) capacities. The significance of past capacities is almost entirely legal. Forensic psychiatrists are called on to evaluate the defendant's capacity for choice at a time when he or she committed a crime (the insanity defense) and sometimes to speculate about the competence of a deceased person at a time in the past when he or she made a will. More rarely, forensic psychiatrists deal with retrospective capacities to manage affairs or to make contracts. None of these interesting, but primarily forensic, issues are discussed here.

The assessment of present or contemporaneous capacities usually involves an evaluation of the patient's capacity to choose. Patients have the opportunity to make a number of choices related to their treatment and to the management of their affairs. Their freedom to choose, however, may be compromised if they lack certain mental capacities that are essential for making adaptive or self-serving choices. Delirious patients, for example, cannot make rational choices with regard to their treatment. Paranoid schizophrenic patients may lack the capacity to make a rational choice about their need for hospitalization. Demented or manic patients are unlikely to have the capacity to make appropriate economic decisions.

The assessment of the capacity to choose may have legal as well as clinical implications. Some patients elect to refuse a psychiatric or medical treatment when such a choice seems to be against their best interest; before they can be treated without consent, they must be determined to be incompetent (i.e., lacking the capacity to choose). In most jurisdictions, the patient's lack of capacity to choose hospitalization is not a legal criterion for civil commitment. Many psychiatrists, however, believe that such an incapacity should be one of the major criteria for involuntary hospitalization. Finally, patients who cannot make self-protective choices in managing their financial affairs may need to have a legal guardian appointed to take over this function.

The evaluation of capacities to choose brings the psychiatrist into frequent contact with the legal system; at the same time, such an evaluation can hardly be viewed as the exclusive province of the forensic psychiatrist. Even beginning residents who work with psychiatric inpatients must regularly deal with the issue of involuntary commitment and with patients who make seemingly incompetent decisions to refuse treatment. In providing consultation to medical services, psychiatric residents must also make determinations about the competence of delirious, demented, or psychotic patients to accept or refuse treatment.

Future or prospective evaluations of capacities can be viewed as predictions, that is, statements about how the patient is likely to respond to a variety of tasks imposed by different environments. When the physician makes recommendations about whether the hospitalized patient should receive occupational therapy, should be allowed off the ward, should have a roommate, should participate in a family conference, or should have visitors, the doctor tries to determine whether the patient has the capacity to meet the demands of the new situation without experiencing adverse behavioral or experiential consequences. As a rule, in making this kind of evaluation, it is the behavioral consequences (i.e., the patient's capacity to deal with situations without acting in a deviant or socially unacceptable manner) that are given the most weight. It is also important, however, to consider the patient's capacity to deal with new situations without experiencing too many painful emotions. Patients may not do anything inappropriate during a family conference, but their participation may lead to their becoming more depressed and anxious if they do not have the capacity to cope with the stress of the conference.

Decisions involving the activities of hospitalized patients deal primarily with the near future and require the evaluation of short-term consequences. Here, the patient is usually regarded as unable to make such decisions without guidance and is accordingly advised or directed by the physician. However, if the patient is to be sent home on a pass or is to be discharged, there may also be concern about later consequences and about the patient's longer term capacities. By the time the patient is ready to leave the hospital, he or she has presumably recovered sufficient capacity to choose so as to be able to participate in the ultimate decision. In this situation, the clinician must evaluate the patient's capacity to meet the demands of a totally new environment, a situation where he or she will remain for a considerable period of time. This very critical decision, which is fraught with malpractice implications, is generally left to first-year residents.

In the outpatient setting, the physician usually helps the patient decide whether to work, to enter into new relationships, to modify various living arrangements, or to enter the hospital. Here, if the patient's assessment of his or her capacities appears to be accurate, the physician may not even provide advice about future activity but may merely help the patient weigh his or her options.

Prospective evaluations of capacity have potential moral consequences. These are determined by the extent to which the physician's recommendation either excuses or fails to excuse the patient from an obligation. Patients may be told that they are capable of returning to work and may be advised to do so. If they elect not to work, they may, in effect, be judged blameworthy (by themselves and others) for having failed to perform an obligation. On the other hand, patients advised that they currently lack the capacity to work are excused from that obligation. They will not be blamed for their inactivity by society, their families, or themselves.

HOW DOES THE CLINICIAN EVALUATE THE PATIENT'S CAPACITY TO MAKE DECISIONS OR TO CHOOSE?

One immediate moral or legal problem in evaluating the capacity to choose is determining what standard will be used to judge whether the patient's choice is "right." Up to now, I have used words like *adaptive* or *appropriate* in describing the standards for evaluating choice, but these terms are hardly satisfactory. The determination of what is an adaptive choice for a given individual depends a great deal on value judgments; in effect, these are decisions that someone else must make about what is best for that person. The term *appropriate* has similar problems and, in addition, does not account for situations in which altruistic motivations influence choice. (A perfectly rational person may decline a potentially helpful medical procedure in order to save his or her family the expense, or a highly religious person may refuse a treatment such as a blood transfusion even if this refusal increases his or her risk of suffering and death.) Nor is the problem solved by arguing that the standard should be "what is in the patient's best interest." Value preferences usually influence judgments of what is best for anyone, and well-meaning people come out on different sides of this question.

Philosophers and jurists have dealt with the question of the "right" choice for the patient by focusing on the issue of individual autonomy. They have developed a doctrine called *substitute judgment*, which directs the court to consider how an incompetent person *would* have chosen if he or she were actually competent. Such a choice need not be compatible with what would appear to be the patient's immediate "best interest." The details of this doctrine need not be spelled out here, except to note that this approach still requires the courts to infer what the competent patient *would* have wanted. Often, they have used their own perception of what is "right" in making this determination.

All of the above concerns have clinical as well as legal implications. Clinicians are often alerted to the existence of impaired capacities when the patient appears to be making an "irrational" choice. They are tempted to judge the rightness of the patient's choice by applying their own value systems; in brief, they assume that the right or rational choice is the choice that they themselves would have made. Thus, physicians rarely question the competence of patients who do what they are advised to do, even when these patients are severely impaired. The patients' capacities are questioned by physicians only when the patients refuse to make the choices that the physicians view as the right ones.

Because it is often unclear what is right, the clinician should not make too many inferences about the patient's capacities based on the rationality of the patient's choice. This should be the rule even when the patient consents to treatment. When a highly disturbed patient provides what seems to be a rational consent to treatment, the physician should at least consider whether that consent is a competent one. When a patient refuses to follow medical advice, the physician should not automatically assume incompetency but should consider the possibility that the patient has good reasons for coming to that decision.

The physician's concern with the "rightness" of the patient's choice is understandable. The observation that the patient is making a clearly maladaptive choice is what usually leads the doctor to suspect that the patient may have some type of mental impairment. *Ultimately, however, the clinician cannot judge capacity to choose by focusing on the quality of the choice.* Instead, the clinician must examine the intactness of the mental processes that the patient uses in making that choice. This approach allows the clinician to work within the confines of his or her expertise and, at least temporarily, to avoid a preoccupation with the social and moral consequences of the patient's decision.

Often, but certainly not always, choices that appear to be maladaptive or irrational are based on mental impairments. In these cases, either on his or her own or with the assistance of legal agencies, the physician will try to override the patient's choice. In many jurisdictions, the physician does not have to invoke legal sanctions to provide medical treatment to those who do not consent. The doctor simply informs family members of the patient's lack of capacity, and the family members' consent is then sufficient. The physician who finds no mental impairments that account for a maladaptive choice should *play no part* in attempting to override that choice. Commonly, the physician encounters situations in which impairments are moderate, and it is not entirely clear how they have led to an apparently maladaptive choice. Here, the consent of the family may not be sufficient. If there appear to be strong moral or social reasons for overriding a maladaptive choice, the physician advises family members or legal agencies about the possible treatment choices and about how the patient's impairments may preclude effective decision making. The courts then decide what should be done.

An additional complexity in assessing the capacity to choose is that mental impairments may compromise a patient's capacity to make some choices but not others. For example, a patient who believes that his physicians are trying to poison him may be impaired in his capacity to choose to refuse medication. He may have full capacity, however, to choose how to spend his money. Therefore, it is necessary for the physician to begin an evaluation of the patient's capacity to choose by first defining what choices the patient is dealing with. For example, these may range from taking neuroleptic medication to entering the hospital or spending one's last dollar on a Rolls Royce. The physician then restricts himself or herself to assessing capacities to make that specific choice.

Once the precise nature of the choice is ascertained, the clinician should make an objective review of its possible benefits and risks and what alternative choices are available. In assessing the patient's capacity to refuse medication, for example, the physician will want to know the possible benefits of the drug in question, all side effects and risks, the availability of alternative treatments, and what is likely to happen if the patient receives no treatment. Once the clinician is fully aware of the benefits of, the risks of, and the alternatives to the choice in question, the clinician must make sure that this information is communicated to the patient as completely and clearly as possible. It is much easier to evaluate the intactness of those mental processes involved in making a choice if the patient has full knowledge of the possible consequences of that choice. (Ordinarily, the physician will want to make sure that the patient has heard this information even when that patient's capacity is not being evaluated. The legal and ethical doctrine of informed consent is based on the idea that patients cannot make appropriate choices without having as much knowledge as possible about the consequences of each choice. A full disclosure of information enhances the patient's sense of autonomy and communicates the physician's attitude of respect. Such disclosure may make the patient more willing to cooperate with the physician's recommendations.)

Once the benefits, risks, and alternatives of possible choices are communicated, the clinician's task is to determine if the patient has perceived them correctly. Patients who are disoriented, who cannot sustain attention, who have receptive aphasia, who are preoccupied with disturbing thoughts, or who are distracted by hallucinations may not accurately perceive what the clinician tells them. They may have difficulty in making the "right" choice because they lack access to information about the consequences of their choices. Ordinarily, the clinician can obtain a rough gauge of the presence of some perceptual difficulty by simply asking the patient to repeat what he or she has been told about benefits, risks, and alternatives.

The clinician should then consider whether the patient has any impairments that would interfere with an intellectual understanding of the choices involved. Here, limitations in intelligence are important. A patient may carefully attend when the doctor tells him that there is a 10% chance of serious complications, but if he does not understand percentages, this communication is of little help in making a decision. Deficits of recent memory may also preclude rational understanding. The patient who quickly forgets possible benefits or risks cannot be said to have sufficient understanding to make an adaptive or appropriate choice.

The next step involves examining aspects of the patterns of the patient's thinking, especially the content of thought, that may lead to a distorted evaluation (either by exaggeration or by minimization) of risks, benefits, or alternatives. A disturbed patient who believes that he is being poisoned, for example, may exaggerate the risks of taking oral medication. A patient who believes that she has been designated by God to suffer may view a slow-acting nonpharmaceutical treatment as more desirable than medication. Generally, the kind of irrational thinking that results in treatment refusal involves delusional ideas; these, in turn, lead the patient to exaggerate risks or minimize benefits.

Some patients distort risks and benefits on the basis of patterns of thought that do not rise to the level of delusional thinking. Learned prejudices or fears relating to such issues as hospitalization or submitting to medical procedures may encourage the patient to make choices that are less than adaptive. Here, the clinician may be on shaky ground in assessing capacity. Idiosyncratic belief systems, especially those based on religious convictions or on a belief in nonmedical aspects of healing, should not be viewed unreflectively as irrational.

The clinician next considers how emotional states may be involved in the distortion of risks, benefits, or alternatives. Patients who are depressed are likely to minimize both the benefits and the risks of treatment, although they may also exaggerate the risks. Anxious patients are likely to exaggerate the risks. Euphoric patients may exaggerate the benefits and minimize the risks. In making this kind of assessment, the clinician must first identify the patient's predominant emotional states and then try to infer how such emotions may influence his or her choice. The patient's direct statements about how feelings may be influencing his or her choice usually help the clinician to make this inference.

Emotions and the content of thought are often linked. That is certainly the case when the emotion of sadness is associated with thoughts of hopelessness. It is also true in some anxiety disorders, such as phobias, where the patient develops troubling patterns of thinking about feared situations. The physician will also wish to explore how thoughts related to emotional states influence choice. Depressed patients may have patterns of thinking that lead them to minimize the effectiveness of treatment. Because they so much wish to avoid a painful emotional experience, phobic patients may make decisions that do not seem rational to others. A patient who is phobic about flying may choose to take a train across country, a decision that seem irrational to most of us, but that may be the least painful course for that person. Here, a fear of encountering a painful emotional state limits the acceptable choices available to the patient.

Finally, the clinician assesses the patient's capacity to measure the risks of benefits of a particular choice against the risks and benefits of alternative choices. Such measurement requires that the patient be able to consider a number of issues at the same time, to assess how various benefits and risks may meet his or her perceived needs or may influence her or his life, and to place a personal value on each risk or benefit. The patient must then be able to sum up factors symbolically on the benefit and the risk side of the decision-making task. Finally, the patient must have a capacity for abstract thinking that allows the projection of himself or herself into the future and an evaluation of how he or she will be influenced by various outcomes. These are all complex cognitive functions that can be compromised by organic brain disease and/or by the thought disorder associated with a major psychosis.

In summary, the steps involved in assessing capacity to choose are:

1. Determining exactly what choice the patient is being asked to make.
2. Ascertaining the risks and benefits of a particular choice and the alternatives.
3. Fully communicating risks, benefits, and alternatives to the patient.
4. Assessing whether the patient has perceived the information provided.
5. Assessing whether the patient understands the information provided.
6. Determining if there are disturbances of emotionality or thinking that lead to distortion in the risk–benefit–alternative assessment.
7. Assessing the patient's capacity to weigh alternatives.

It should be emphasized that the data needed to make assessments 1 through 7 are obtained in the process of evaluating the patient's mental status.

HOW DOES THE CLINICIAN EVALUATE THE PATIENT'S CAPACITY TO RESPOND ADAPTIVELY TO FUTURE ENVIRONMENTS?

The capacity to respond to future environments is the patient's ability to meet environmental expectations without behaving deviantly or experiencing excessive suffering. Essentially, this is an evaluation of the patient's capacity to perform a task successfully. Such an evaluation has two major components: first, the patient's capacity actually to perform the behavioral requirements of the task and, second, the patient's capacity to perform the task successfully, that is, without being disruptive and without experiencing serious suffering or distress. These two components are obviously interrelated. Poor performance increases the risk of disruptiveness or distress, and disruptive behavior or distress interferes with performance. In spite of the interrelatedness of these two aspects of prospective capacity, it is useful to consider them separately.

The clinician begins the evaluation of the capacity to perform a task by asking, "What does the task require or what will be expected of the patient in the particular environment to which he or she will be exposed?" Depressed patients who are asked to leave their rooms and to spend time in the day room can probably meet the environmental expectations by just sitting quietly. If they watch TV with interest or communicate with other patients or staff, they are, of course, meeting a higher level of expectation. But these patients would still be judged as having the capacity to leave their rooms if they simply were not disruptive or in greater than usual distress while in the day room. Patients who are asked to attend a family conference are exposed to a higher level of expectations. They will be expected to understand at least some of what is being said and may also be asked to communicate with others. Environmental expectations become ever greater in work situations. Here, the patient may need a variety of intellectual and/or motor skills or, in some cases, good communicative skills.

The clinician's second task is to determine what mental skills are required if the patient is to meet the demands of a particular task. In most of the environments in which the patient is expected to interact nondisruptively with others, or to perform some intellectual or manual task, the patient will need some ability to attend to the task and to concentrate on it. It is also critical that the patient's perceptual functioning be sufficiently intact so that he or she understands what is expected of him or her. Most complex environments also require the patient to have communicative skills. Any disorder in the patient's thinking or any expressive language disorder may impair the patient's performance.

The third step in the evaluation of prospective capacity is to determine if the patient has the mental skills that the task requires and is free of mental impairments that would compromise his or her performance. Here, the clinician first determines if the patient has sufficient perceptual, intellectual, and communicative skills to perform the task. This information is generally obtained from the mental status examination. The clinician then tries to determine if there are disturbances in emotionality or thinking that may impair performance. Again, the clinician turns to the mental status examination and estimates how any abnormalities noted, such as delusions, hallucinations, or painful emotional states, may compromise the patient's success in meeting a particular environmental task.

It is useful to assume that, as long as the patient is succeeding in the behavioral aspects of a task, he or she will suffer less and will refrain from exhibiting disruptive behavior. This means that the clinician who advises the patient to take on a given task should have a high expectation that the patient has the perceptual, cognitive, and emotional competencies requisite for mastering it. If the patient senses failure of mastery, he or she will experience emotional distress. If those in the environment note the patient's failure, they may do things to increase the stress levels and thus put the patient at more risk of emotional distress or disruptive behavior.

Having considered the patient's perceptual, cognitive, and emotional capacities to accomplish a task or to meet environmental expectations, the clinician then proceeds to assess the likely extent of the patient's suffering or the probability of the patient's behaving disruptively if he or she attempts to perform that task. These are really predictions, and they are very difficult to make. First of all, it is hard to know how much the patient suffers. The degree of distress is not objectively measurable and must often be inferred from the patient's communications and behavior. It is also difficult to determine what degree of suffering that the patient is likely to endure, and at what point we should humanely prevent the patient from taking on a particular task. *In actual practice, clinicians rely primarily on behavioral cues, in particular, the appearance of disruptive or inappropriate behavior, as an indication that suffering is excessive.* This means that prospective capacity is, in large part, measured behaviorally. The patient who accomplishes a task only at the expense of experiencing great agony, but who is not disruptive in response to that agony, is often viewed as competent to deal with that task.

Nevertheless, in clinical work, compassion often dictates protecting patients from tasks that they can accomplish only at the expense of great suffering. Most clinicians would not force an agoraphobic patient to enter a feared environment, even if the patient were judged capable of doing so without acting disruptively. Few clinicians would subject a seriously depressed patient to a stressful interview, even if the patient were unlikely to respond to it with disruptive behavior. Clinicians try to estimate the probable degree of patients' suffering both by considering the patients' capacity to succeed at the task that the environment calls for (an evaluation already described) and by obtaining historical data about how the patients have responded to similar environments in the past. In particular, how have they responded when they have had impairments similar to those that they have now? Much subjective judgment is required here. It is often difficult to uncover a history of the patient undertaking tasks in the past that are similar to current tasks and that the patient undertook while experiencing a similar level of impairment. The reliability with which the patient can report experiential phenomena must also be considered. The clinician can increase the accuracy of this assessment by asking patients for their own prediction of their probable degree of suffering if they take on a particular task. Questions such as "Can you handle this pass without getting upset?" or "How much anxiety do you think you'll have if you decide to go to the hospital party?" or

"Do you worry about having another panic attack if you go shopping?" are helpful.

The clinician finally turns.to the issue of predicting the likelihood that the patient will be disruptive. Here, again, the clinician begins with an assessment of the patient's actual capacity to perform the task. The assumption is that disruptive, noxious, or violent behavior may be a manifestation of insufficient capacity to master the assigned task. Clinicians usually protect against patients' encountering environments in which they are likely to be disruptive, both for the patients' sake and to protect others in that environment.

Once it is ascertained that the patient has the mental capacities to succeed at a task, the clinician relies heavily on the history taking to evaluate the patient's potential disruptiveness. Where there is already a history of disruptiveness occurring in similar environments, that patient is more likely to be disruptive. The likelihood increases if the patient's mental state at the time of the earlier disturbance was similar to his or her present condition. This is true even in dissimilar environments because some disruptive behaviors are learned responses to stress; they are therefore likely to appear in a variety of different circumstances once these are perceived as stressful.

The severity of the disruptiveness may also be related to certain demographic characteristics, such as age or sex. A violent response, for example, is more likely in youthful males. An elderly woman may be less capable of violent acts and is more likely to behave inappropriately in nonviolent ways. Other demographic variables, such as race, education, marital status, or socioeconomic class, help a little in predicting the probability of the forms of disruptiveness characterized as violent.

Often, the patient's actual behavior during the interview will help predict the short-term probability of disruptive conduct. The patient who is pacing the floor, speaking in a loud voice, and making threats is predictably at high risk of doing something disruptive in the near future. The patient's own motivations or predictions regarding future conduct as revealed by his or her statements are also important. When the patient communicates the intent of future disruptiveness, such conduct is more likely to occur.

In making a prediction of disruptive behavior, even in the near future, the clinician must be aware of the limits of accuracy in predicting behavioral events. Certainty is almost never possible. As a rule, the clinician can estimate only the probability that a disruptive event will occur. This estimate must usually be qualified by a consideration of how the environment may respond to and influence the patient. For example, the clinician may estimate that there is a 50 percent chance that a rebellious teenager will storm out of a family conference if his parents persist in their usual pattern of nagging him. This probability may be reduced to zero if the family should behave in a more supportive manner. In all instances, the estimate of potential disruptiveness is most likely to be accurate if the environmental contingencies are also predictable. This means that the clinician's estimate of the patient's capacity to deal with a given task without disruptiveness will also be influenced by an assessment of the nature and the constancy of the environment in which the task is addressed.

The patient's capacity to refrain from disruptive behavior can also be evaluated as an issue of choice. Ordinarily, we assume that behavior, whether conforming or disruptive, is chosen. This is true even when we acknowledge that mental handicaps diminish the range or ease of choice. If disruptive behavior is viewed as an issue of choice, then one has a way to gain some perspective on the patient's capacity to make a future choice to refrain from disruptive conduct. One needs merely to make a type of assessment similar to that used in determining the patient's capacity to make current or contemporaneous choices. The difference here is that the capacity for contemporaneous choice can be estimated on the basis of the patient's current mental status. Estimations of future capacity for choice require an additional judgment: Will the patient's mental status change, both with the passage of time and as he or she moves into different environments?

In this situation, knowledge of the patient's diagnosis may help. To the extent that the diagnosis implies something about the patient's future mental status, it tells something about his or her future capacities. A diagnosis of schizophrenia, for example, suggests a greater likelihood than does a diagnosis of depression that various mental aberrations will still be present in the future.

The prospective evaluation of the capacity to refrain from disruptive conduct, viewed as a matter of choice, begins with a careful consideration of the situation in which disruptiveness is a likely option. For the severely disturbed patient, of course, this can be almost any situation. For less disturbed patients, the most critical situations are those that have elicited disruptiveness in the past or that are likely to be highly stressful. The clinician then evaluates any abnormalities that the patient currently demonstrates and any problems that would impair his or her ability to perceive and understand the risks and benefits of disruptive and nondisruptive responses to a particular situation. This evaluation is followed by a consideration of any disturbed thinking or emotionality that may favor an exaggeration of the benefits of disruptiveness or a minimization of its risks. Delusional ideas of persecution may, for example, lead the patient to believe that disruptiveness is appropriate. Delusional ideas of grandiosity or feelings of elation may lead to an inappropriate minimization of the risks associated with disruptive behavior.

Finally, the clinician considers the patient's capacity to conceptualize and weigh the consequences of disruptive and nondisruptive behavior. Again, it is important to keep in mind that all these assessments are directed to predicting future consequences. Such predictions are based on the assumption that the same mental status aberrations that the clinician observes at the time of the evaluation are likely to be present at the time when a disruptive act is chosen.

In viewing disruptiveness as an issue of choice, personality variables (particularly those that influence the patient's judgment about the consequences of disruptiveness) are often important. Here, the failure to perceive one's actions as others might perceive them and the lack of an ability to empathize with the probable feelings and thoughts of others may be especially critical. The patient who lacks such qualities is handicapped in the capacity to make reasonable predictions about the consequences of his or her being conforming or disruptive. Because the patient does not fully appreciate how others will respond and therefore cannot perceive the full risks of such conduct, she or he is likely to make erroneous judgments about the value of disruptive versus nondisruptive behavior.

In summary, the clinician evaluates prospective capacities by considering, first, whether the patient has the abilities actually to master the task and, second, whether he or she can do so without experiencing undue stress or behaving in a disruptive manner.

The first part of the evaluation involves the following steps:

1. Determining the exact nature of the task to be performed. This will also involve an assessment of the demands of the environment in which it is performed.
2. Determining what skills are required for performance.
3. Determining whether the patient has the requisite skills and is free from impairments that will compromise performance.

The second part of the evaluation is influenced by the results of the first part. It deals with two qualifications: that performance not be too distressing to the patient and that it not be associated with disruptiveness. In addition, the evaluation involves the following steps:

1. Determining by the history and the patient's own predictions whether the patient is likely to experience unusual distress if the task is attempted.
2. Determining by the history, the demographics, the patient's current behavior, his or her own predictions, his or her motivations regarding his or her future behavior, and sometimes his or her diagnosis whether disruptiveness may be reasonably predicted.
3. Assessing the probable environmental contingencies that will favor or diminish disruptiveness.

4. Viewing the patient's possible disruptiveness as an issue of choice. This leads to the use of models for current or contemporaneous choice. These, in turn, allow one to speculate about how current impairments may influence the patient's capacity to choose nondisruptive conduct in some future or prospective situation. This evaluation requires a prediction of whether the patient's current mental status will remain constant or will change. The patient's diagnosis may help the clinician make this prediction.

WHAT ARE SOME EXAMPLES OF HOW PROSPECTIVE ASSESSMENTS OF CAPACITY CAN BE MADE?

The evaluation of prospective capacity is complicated; it may therefore be useful to consider examples of clinical situations in which such evaluations are made. Two of the commonest assessments that confront the beginning student are the estimation of dangerousness to others and the determination of possible suicidality. These assessments have been alluded to in previous chapters. They are important enough, however, so that they will be considered again, this time in terms of the concept of capacities.

In assessing a patient's dangerousness to others, the student must first of all be aware of certain legal traps. The term *dangerousness* has no medical meaning. It is a legal concept designed to indicate potentiality for harmfulness. It is assumed that there is a threshold of potential harmfulness, above which societal actions such as civil commitment may be justified. The use of the term is usually based on that belief. When a court says someone is dangerous, it means that it views that individual's risk of committing harm as high enough so that some societal action to prevent that harm is justifiable. For the physician, the pitfall here is that the law never states what *probability* of what *harm's* occurring in what *time period* is sufficient to justify using the label *dangerous*. Yet, most state statutes require the psychiatrist (who is often the first-year resident) to predict dangerousness.

Obviously, the psychiatrist cannot fulfill this mandate. No professional can determine what the court will consider dangerous; one can only describe and study specific disruptive behaviors that are likely to be harmful to others. Based on these data, one must then try to predict the probability of such behaviors occurring in a given time period and in various environments. Many authors have described the difficulty of this task, and some view it as impossible. Nevertheless, it is one that has been thrust on the psychiatric profession, it has been tacitly accepted by the psychiatric community, and it is one that psychiatrists must therefore do to the best of their ability.

Let us assume that the psychiatrist has been treating a hospitalized patient with a diagnosis of paranoid schizophrenia. Now the time has come to make a decision about whether the patient can be discharged to return to live with his family. It happens that, for years, this patient has experienced unpleasant hallucinations that are associated with his being alternately agitated and depressed. When agitated, the patient tends to be physically assaultive toward his wife and children. He has now been hospitalized for two weeks and has been put on a substantial dose of haloperidol. The physician knows from the patient's history that, as long as he remains on this medication, there is little risk of violent disruptiveness. When the patient stops the medication, however, his symptoms generally escalate and the risk of violence increases.

In trying to decide whether to discharge this patient, one of the first things the physician will think about is what the patient will have to accomplish outside the hospital. In the hospital, few interpersonal or occupational demands have been made on the patient. Once the patient leaves the hospital, he may return to work, and in any case, he must interact with his family and others. Before deciding whether the patient can be discharged, the clinician must determine, first, what skills this patient must have acquired in order to master the task of living outside the hospital, then whether the patient has indeed learned these skills, and, finally, whether the patient is free of impairments that might compromise his performance.

Once it is ascertained that the patient has the mental capacities to perform the task implicit in living outside the hospital, the clinician tries to determine if he is likely to experience unusual distress or disruptiveness when he leaves the hospital. This is ascertained both by reviewing the history with particular emphasis on past episodes of disruptiveness and by the patient's predictions of his own future conduct. Here, the history of the patient's compliance with medication and his own statements about whether he will continue to take the medication are quite important. Equally important issues are whether there is a history of substance abuse, whether the patient has been violent when inebriated, and the patient's current likelihood of abstaining from nonprescribed drugs.

The clinician next assesses various aspects of the environment that the patient will encounter that may favor or diminish disruptiveness. Here, the attitude his employer, his spouse, and other family members have may be extremely important. This attitude may be supportive or abrasive; to the extent that the clinician is aware of the supportiveness or lack of supportiveness of significant variables in the patient's environment, he will make a more accurate prediction. If, for example, the wife does not remind the patient to take his medication or is unsympathetic and callous toward disabilities related to the patient's illness, the risk of disruptiveness is much greater.

Finally, the physician can view the patient's possible disruptiveness as an issue of choice. This view requires some speculation about what the individual's mental status is likely to be in the face of various contingencies. Knowing that this particular patient has a diagnosis of paranoid schizophrenia, the physician may assume that, if he stops taking his medication or is exposed to unusual stress, various impairments will compromise his ability to weigh risks, benefits, and alternative actions.

An easier scenario involves a patient with a dual diagnosis of schizophrenic disorder and antisocial personality disorder who has just assaulted his wife and broken her jaw. In this instance, the physician is examining that patient in the emergency room to determine whether involuntary commitment is necessary. Here, the clinician is obviously concerned about violent disruptiveness.

In order to be certain that the patient's violence is related to his mental illness and is not simply an isolated event, the clinician will want to determine the quality of the patient's functioning in the most recent environment. In particular, the doctor will want to know how the patient has been getting along with individuals other than his wife, and whether the patient has been able to work. The doctor will try to determine whether there are situations in which the patient lacked the skills necessary for proper performance or suffered from impairments that compromised his performance.

The clinician then tries to speculate whether, if he is not hospitalized, the patient will continue to experience unusual distress or will become disruptive. In determining the likelihood of future violence, the clinician relies on the patient's history, demographics, current behavior, predictions, and apparent motivations with regard to his future behavior. The clinician also assesses the probable environmental contingencies that would either favor or diminish disruptiveness. Here, the attitude of the wife and of other significant people in the environment would be extremely important.

Finally, the clinician views the patient's disruptiveness as an issue of choice and looks for various aberrations in the mental status examination that may compromise the patient's capacity to make risk–benefit determinations. Because the clinician is concerned only about the prediction of short-term events in this type of situation, he is likely to assume that any incapacities revealed in the emergency room will also be present in the near future. Because this assumption is usually justified, the accuracy of evaluation of short-term dangerousness is likely to be greater than evaluation of long-term dangerousness.

A third example of prospective capacity evaluation is the decision of whether to hospitalize an outpatient who is threatening suicide. Here, the clinician begins with an assessment of what the patient needs to do in his or her current occupational and interpersonal environment and asks what skills are required for performance, and whether the patient has the requisite skills and is free of impairments that may compromise performance. This assessment is especially important with suicidal patients, as failure to master any task assigned to them generally deepens their level of depression and increases the risk of suicide. The clinician then turns to evaluating the extent of the patient's suicidal motivation, that is, whether the patient is simply thinking about suicide or is actively contemplating it, how he or she plans to do it, and whether he or she has the means to do it. The history of previous suicidal behavior, the history of substance abuse, demographics (variables such as age, sex, marital status, and religion have at least some relation to suicide), and the patient's level of current emotional distress or suffering can then be evaluated.

The clinician next turns to the possible environmental contingencies that will influence the probability of suicide. It is important to determine whether there are supportive figures in the environment or whether the environment will continue to be stressful. The doctor also tries to determine whether there will be people available to be with the patient and to monitor his or her behavior, or whether the patient will be alone. The clinician must also inquire about whether the patient has the means for undertaking a suicidal act.

Finally, the clinician views the patient's potential suicide as an issue of choice and looks at various impairments, particularly the existence of depression, that may influence both the patient's capacity to evaluate the risks, benefits, and alternatives of suicide and the patient's ability to refrain from this type of behavior.

The above examples are common enough and are certainly among the most troubling prospective assessments that beginning psychiatrists must make. However, the same type of conceptualization is involved in making prospective assessments of the patient's day-to-day capacities, such as those involved in leaving the ward, attending a family conference, or taking on some new work-related task. Again, the clinician begins by looking at the patient's capacity actually to perform the task. The clinician then considers the various psychiatric impairments and environmental contingencies that would increase the patient's suffering or increase the likelihood of disruptive behavior if he or she undertakes that task.

A FINAL NOTE ON EVALUATION OF CAPACITIES

The material presented in this chapter is largely based on my experiences in forensic psychiatry, a subspecialty that deals almost exclusively with the evaluation of capacities. Even in forensic psychiatry, however, evaluation has not been systematically conceptualized as a capacity issue and there are few published guidelines for capacity evaluation. Only recently has there been a general consensus in forensic psychiatry that such conceptualization is a critical need of that specialty.

After struggling through this chapter, the reader may wonder as to the relevance of capacity evaluation to nonforensic psychiatric patients. Why include this admittedly difficult material in a book subtitled, *A Primer*? I decided to include it because I believe that capacity evaluation is an inherent part of psychiatric practice. As long as abnormal behavior is a major criteria in the definition of most mental disorders, the clinician must be concerned with estimating current capacities and predicting future capacities of patients' behavior including their capacity to refrain from behaving in certain ways. It also seems likely that our society will increasingly call upon psychiatrists to describe, quantify, and predict behavioral manifestations of illness. Although our tools for evaluating capacities, especially future capacities, may be primitive, it is critical that psychiatrists, and beginners as well, have some conceptual framework for thinking about this issue.

FOR FURTHER READING

Appelbaum, P. S., and Grisso, T. Assessing patients' capacities to consent to treatment. *New England Journal of Medicine*, 319–25, 1635–1538, December, 1988.

Drane, J. F. The many faces of competency. *Hastings Center Report*, 15(2): 17–21, 1985.

Grisso, T. *Evaluating competence: Forensic assessments and instruments*. New York, Plenum, 1986.

Monahan, N. The prediction of violent behavior: Toward a second generation of theory and policy. *American Journal of Psychiatry*, 141:10–15, 1984.

Index

2